Painkillers
Prescription Dependency

ILLICIT AND MISUSED DRUGS

ILLICIT AND MISUSED DRUGS

Painkillers
Prescription Dependency

By Ida Walker

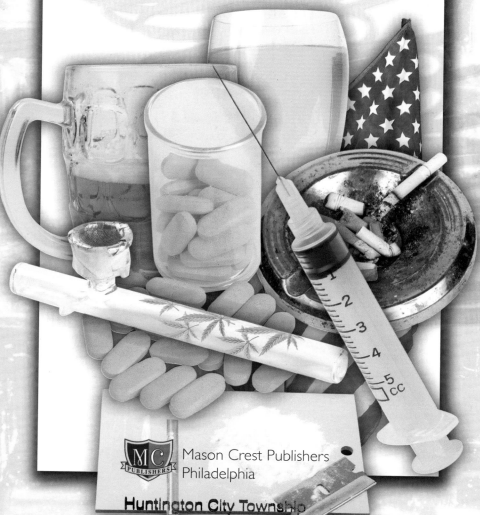

Mason Crest Publishers
Philadelphia

Mason Crest Publishers Inc.
370 Reed Road
Broomall, Pennsylvania 19008
(866) MCP-BOOK (toll free)
www.masoncrest.com

First printing
1 2 3 4 5 6 7 8 9 10
Library of Congress Cataloging-in-Publication Data
ISBN-13: 978-1-4222-0149-7 (series)

Walker, Ida.
  Painkillers : prescription dependency / by Ida Walker.
      p. cm. — (Illicit and misused drugs)
  Includes bibliographical references and index.
  ISBN 1-4222-0161-9
  1. Drug addiction. 2. Analgesics. 3. Narcotics. I. Title.
RC566.W35 2008
362.29—dc22
                                        2006023091

Interior design by Benjamin Stewart.
Cover design by MK Bassett-Harvey.
Produced by Harding House Publishing Service Inc.
Vestal, New York.
www.hardinghousepages.com

Cover image design by Peter Spires Culotta.
Cover photography: iStock Photography (Maartje van Caspel,
    Natalia Bratslavsky), Palisade Innovations (Peter Culotta)
Printed in the Hashemite Kingdom of Jordan.

This book is meant to educate and should not be used as an alternative to ap-
propriate medical care. Its creators have made every effort to ensure that the
information presented is accurate—but it is not intended to substitute for the
help and services of trained professionals.

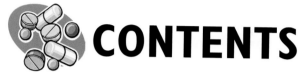# CONTENTS

INTRODUCTION

Addicting drugs are among the greatest challenges to health, well-being, and the sense of independence and freedom for which we all strive—and yet these drugs are present in the everyday lives of most people. Almost every home has alcohol or tobacco waiting to be used, and has medicine cabinets stocked with possibly outdated but still potentially deadly drugs. Almost everyone has a friend or loved one with an addiction-related problem. Almost everyone seems to have a solution neatly summarized by word or phrase: medicalization, legalization, criminalization, war-on-drugs.

For better and for worse, drug information seems to be everywhere, but what information sources can you trust? How do you separate misinformation (whether deliberate or born of ignorance and prejudice) from the facts? Are prescription drugs safer than "street" drugs? Is occasional drug use really harmful? Is cigarette smoking more addictive than heroin? Is marijuana safer than alcohol? Are the harms caused by drug use limited to the users? Can some people become addicted following just a few exposures? Is treatment or counseling just for those with serious addiction problems?

These are just a few of the many questions addressed in this series. It is an empowering series because it provides the information and perspectives that can help people come to their own opinions and find answers to the challenges posed by drugs in their own lives. The series also provides further resources for information and assistance, recognizing that no single source has all the answers. It should be of interest and relevance to areas of study spanning biology, chemistry, history, health, social studies and more. Its efforts to provide a real-world context for the information that is clearly presented but not overly simplified should be appreciated by students, teachers, and parents.

The series is especially commendable in that it does not pretend to pose easy answers or imply that all decisions can be made on the basis of simple facts: some challenges have no immediate or simple solutions, and some solutions will need to rely as much upon basic values as basic facts. Despite this, the series should help to at least provide a foundation of knowledge. In the end, it may help as much by pointing out where the solutions are not simple, obvious, or known to work. In fact, at many points, the reader is challenged to think for him- or herself by being asked what his or her opinion is.

A core concept of the series is to recognize that we will never have all the facts, and many of the decisions will never be easy. Hopefully, however, armed with information, perspective, and resources, readers will be better prepared for taking on the challenges posed by addictive drugs in everyday life.

— *Jack E. Henningfield, Ph.D.*

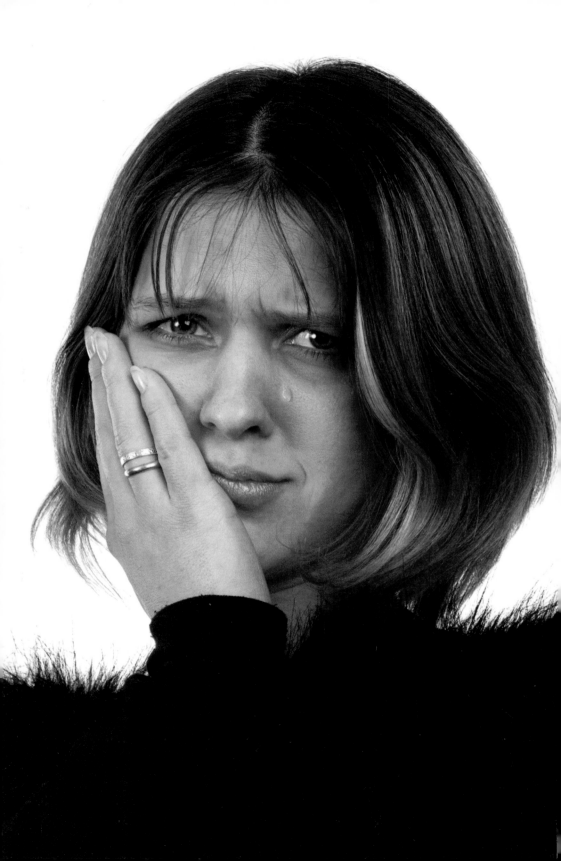

1 What Is Pain?

Pain is a necessary part of human life. It's a warning signal, indicating that something isn't right. It logically follows then, that most people have some form of painkiller in their medicine cabinet. After all, almost everyone has a headache or other assorted ache or pain that needs relief.

For some people, though, physical pain is part of their everyday life. Over-the-counter pain relievers will not work for their pain. For them, prescription painkillers are the most effective way of controlling their pain. To understand how painkillers work, it is necessary to have a basic understanding of what pain is and how the body feels pain.

Definition

First, pain is a broad term for an unpleasant feeling. The International Association for the Study of Pain (IASP)

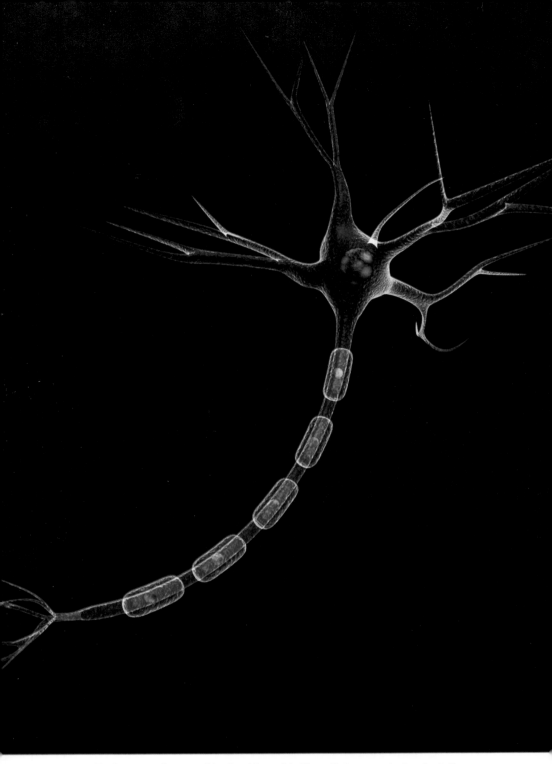

Each neuron has a cell body with a whip-like tail; the strands that look like roots are called dendrites.

differentiates between pain and nociception. According to the IASP, the *neuropsychological* term nociception refers to the transmission of physiological pain along the nerves, whereas the word pain can be understood to mean emotional pain and cannot be *quantified*. However, since most people are familiar with the term pain, in the context of this book, it is used to mean nociception.

How the Body Feels Pain

You stub your toe, and almost immediately, you wince, perhaps yell, and wipe tears from your eyes. You're in pain, and frankly, you probably don't care why—beyond the fact that you hurt your toe.

The body is a complex machine, and the ability to feel pain is just one of its complicated functions. Each of those functions must go through the nervous system in order for a reaction to be processed. The nervous system is made up of the afferent nerve fibers and their receptors, efferent nerve fibers and the muscles and glands, and the central nervous system (CNS), composed of the brain and spinal cord. Almost every inch of the human body is touched by nerve fibers, made up of nerve cells, or neurons. In the case of pain, nociceptors are the nerve endings whose responsibility it is to send the pain impulses indicating that something hurts. These neurons are the messengers responsible for eventually passing along the information to the brain. Each nerve cell consists of an a cell body with an axon, a whip-like tail, at one end and root-looking projections called dendrites at the other end. Nociceptors can be less than a centimeter long or extend more than three feet in length across the synapses, the spaces between nerve endings.

Fast Fact

Some people are born without the ability to feel pain. This condition, called "congenital insensitivity to pain with anhidrosis" (CIPA), is so rare that there are no figures on how many individuals are affected.

Individuals with CIPA have never felt pain. They can often discriminate touch, but not temperature. Persons with CIPA also usually do not sweat, which is what anhidrosis means.

Life can be very difficult for individuals with CIPA, especially for young children. Many bite off the tips of their tongues. Infections, fractured and broken bones, even such conditions as appendicitis can go undetected. Many very young children with this condition suffer corneal damage by simply poking themselves in the eye with a finger. Life expectancy for people with CIPA is often compromised because of their condition.

Afferent and efferent nerve fibers (also called the peripheral nervous system) work together in a carefully designed communication system. The body uses **neurotransmitters** to signal the nearby nerve endings that something has been damaged. These nerve endings use afferent nerve fibers to send out a series of electrochemical impulses first to the spinal cord and then on to the cerebral cortex, the part of the brain responsible for the perception of sensations, learning, reasoning, and memory. Afferent nerve fibers send out the "ouch" message. The efferent nerve fibers send signals from the CNS to the muscles, glands, or organs. These messages spur the body into a reaction to the pain. Using our stubbed toe as an example, the afferent nerve fibers would let the CNS know that there is pain, and the efferent nerve fibers might tell the leg muscle to contract, moving the toe away from the pain source as quickly as possible.

Type of Pain

All pain is not the same. It is classified by how long it lasts and grouped by its source.

Pain can be acute or chronic. By definition, acute pain lasts for a short time or has an easily identifiable cause. Acute pain tells the body that injury or disease, such as cancer, has already occurred. It is generally focused on a particular area, though it can *radiate* to other locations

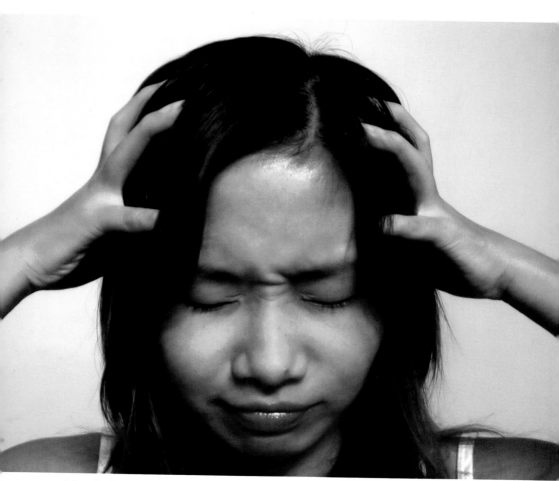

A headache is usually considered to be an acute pain, but in some cases, it can become chronic.

from that site. Acute pain can have a rapid onset or come on more slowly. Many times it begins with a sharp pain, which is then followed by an aching sensation. Acute pain responds well to painkillers.

Chronic pain is long term or frequently recurring, lasting longer than might be expected for the particular type of injury. Treating chronic pain can be more difficult than acute pain. In some chronic pain cases, surgery may even be required for the individual to achieve some relief.

The pain's source is another way medical authorities classify pain. Cutaneous pain comes from injury to the body's superficial tissues. Such injuries would include paper cuts, first-degree burns, and minor lacerations. Because of its nearness to a high number of nociceptors, the pain is localized and generally lasts only a short while.

Neuropathic pain is caused by damage to the nerve tissue. This damage often causes a disruption in the pain messenger system, described earlier in the chapter. The message being sent to the brain may become garbled or misinterpreted, so that it sends out pain signals though there are no physical reasons for the pain.

One of the least understood sources of pain is phantom limb pain. Almost all amputees and **quadriplegics** report some degree of phantom limb pain. With this condition, the individual feels burning or aching coming from a limb that has been amputated or from which nerve signals no longer are sent. In some cases, a less painful condition called phantom limb sensations has been reported by children born without a limb.

Sprains and pain caused by broken bones are examples of somatic pain. Ligaments, tendons, bones, and blood vessels are the sources of this type of pain. Because there

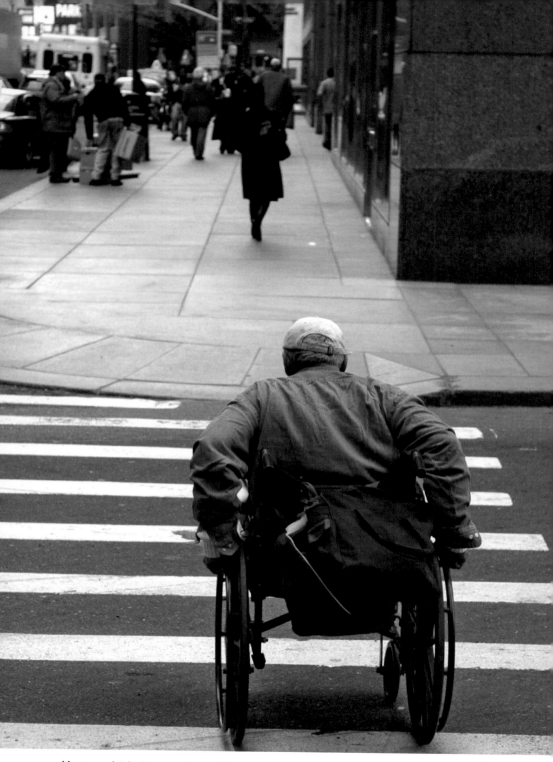

Most quadriplegics experience phantom limb pain, even though nerve signals are no longer being sent by the paralyzed or missing legs.

Painkillers—Prescription Dependency 15

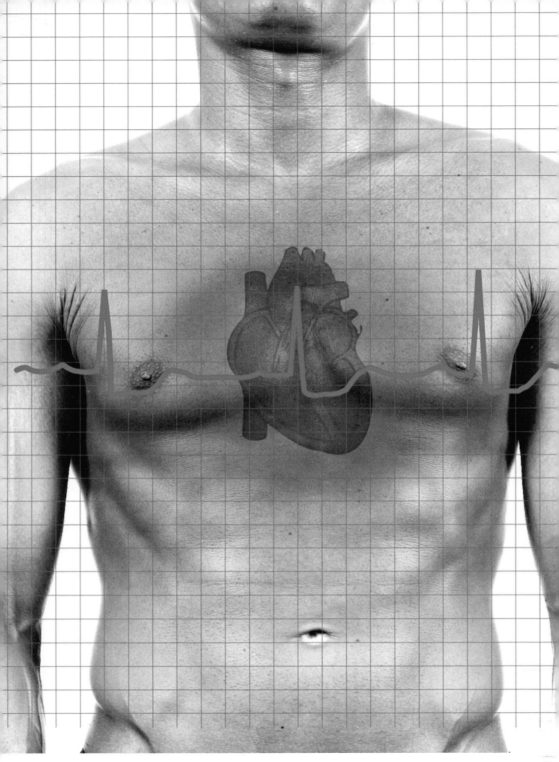

Injury to the heart may be perceived as pain in the shoulder, arm, abdomen, or jaw.

are not many nociceptors in these areas, an aching sensation, more *dispersed* than localized, may be reported by the individual with this type of pain.

Visceral pain comes from the body's internal organs. Because there are even fewer nociceptors in that area than in the sources of somatic pain, the pain in these areas has more of an aching sensation and is longer lasting than somatic pain. Visceral pain can be hard to trace, as tissue injury often results in referred pain, in which an area unrelated to the source of the injury area exhibits the pain. One of the best-known examples of this type of visceral pain is a myocardial infarction—a heart attack. Although the pain-causing injury occurs in the heart, pain may be felt in the left shoulder or arm, abdomen, or jaw. Researchers believe that this referred pain occurs because viscera pain receptors affect the same spinal cord neurons as the cutaneous tissue. The brain usually associates the excitement of these neurons with somatic tissues in the skin or muscles, so it believes the pain actually coming from organs such as the heart is coming from the skin.

Although some pain is good for us—even necessary for survival—most people would rather not be in pain any more than absolutely necessary. Pain is obviously a bad thing.

But human beings haven't always looked at pain that way.

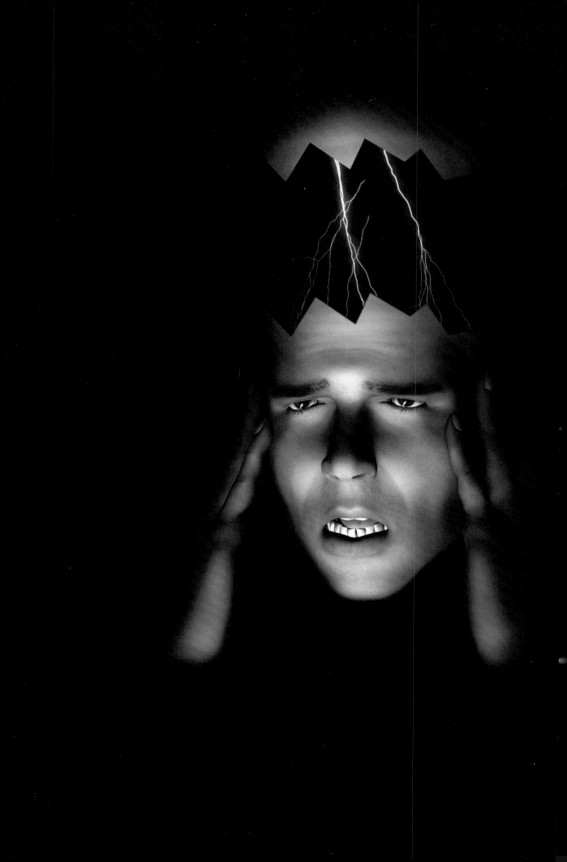

2 The History of Pain

Pain is a universal experience—but at the same time, it is a totally private one as well: no one else can ever truly understand the pain you feel. Doctors and nurses may ask patients to rate their pain on a scale of one to ten—but who's to say that what one person perceives as a five on the pain scale might not be a ten on someone else's scale?

Author David Morris writes in *The Culture of Pain* about the modern **Western** world's perception of this sensation. He points out that in the world where most of us live today, pain is seen mostly as an alarm—an indication that something is wrong in our body that needs to be fixed. But this wasn't always the case. In the past, pain was viewed as a message from God. According to Morris, "Pain had an enormous range of meanings before we shrunk it down to one—meaningless."

A patient brochure at a pain management center states:

Pain is different for everyone. No one else feels your pain as you do. Your ability to live with your pain depends on understanding what causes the pain, your feelings or emotions, and how others react to your pain. Pain is easier to put up with if you are busy, having a good time, or with people you enjoy. The very same pain hurts more when you are not active, feel alone, discouraged, and misunderstood.

Medieval Pain

Pain in the Middle Ages had a powerful spiritual significance. Religion permeated all areas of life, and the suffering Christ was a central image. Artists graphically portrayed the agony of Christ on the cross, as well as the torture of the saints. Agony and ecstasy were often linked in these works, while in other cases, the artists indicated the connection between pain and patience, a resigned acceptance of God's will. For some medieval religious orders, pain was so necessary to mystical revelation that they inflicted pain on themselves.

Meanwhile, Christianity also influenced medieval doctors. They believed that Adam's Fall brought pain to all humanity, so that pain as a punishment for sin was now central to the human experience. People experienced pain because God was disciplining them, the way a parent might discipline a child. As human beings submitted to God's hand on their lives in the form of pain, they grew to be better people, closer to God, less sinful.

However, at the same time, medieval schools of medicine debated the physical causes and characteristics of suffering. They believed that pain occurred when the body's "humors" (blood, phlegm, yellow bile, and black bile) were disrupted. Painkillers were not recommended, since they only masked the pain's cause; instead, doctors worked to restore balance to the body's humors by blood-letting, administering laxatives or **purgatives**, and monitoring food, drink, and sleep.

From the thirteenth century on, however, the medical community was a growing force in Western culture. As medicine developed, the concept of pain also began to change. By the seventeenth century, the French philosopher Rene Descartes had proposed that the human body and the human spirit were two totally separate things; what influenced one had no effect on the other. In his works, he drew a diagram of pain as a mechanized process lacking any social or spiritual meaning; it was simply the result of nerves being stimulated in a particular way.

Assessing Pain

Doctors use several different tools for helping them assess a patient's pain.

- One that is often used with young patients or those with mental impairments is the Wong-Baker Faces Pain Rating Scale. Designed for children aged three years and older, the Wong-Baker Faces Pain Rating Scale offers a visual description for those who don't have the verbal skills to explain how their symptoms make them feel.
- A numerical pain scale allows you to describe the intensity of your discomfort in numbers ranging from 0 (no pain) to 10 (extreme pain). Rating the intensity of sensation is one way of helping your doctor determine treatment. Some researchers believe that this type of combination scale may be most sensitive to gender and ethnic differences in describing pain.
- A verbal pain scale uses these words: no pain, mild pain, moderate pain, severe pain.

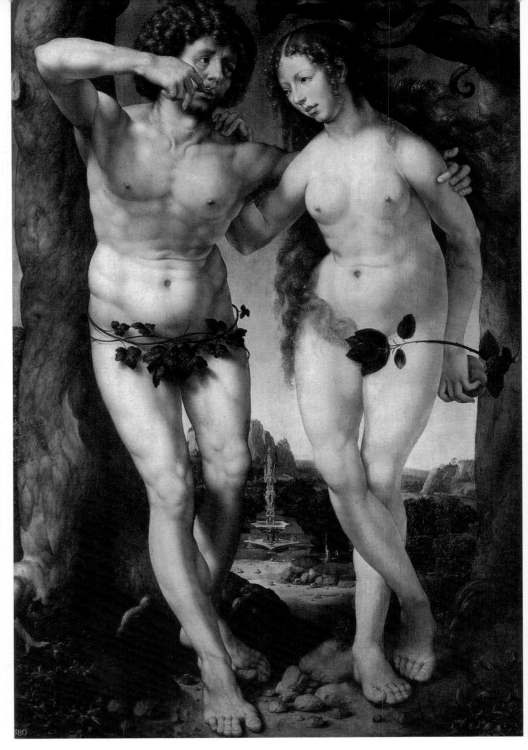

In the sixteenth century, when this painting was created by the artist Jan Gossaert, most people still believed that human pain was the result of Adam and Eve's sin.

22 **Chapter 2—The History of Pain**

Nineteenth-Century Pain

In 1892, the American psychologist William James wrote, "The physiology of pain is still an *enigma*." In other words, the physical basis for pain was as much mystery as ever, despite the growing ability to treat pain with local and general anesthetics. These treatments worked—but doctors didn't know why.

At the same time, Christianity's traditional interpretations of pain were starting to be questioned in new and deeper ways. Westerners were questioning how a loving God could willingly inflict pain on his children. The prestigious medical journal *Lancet* was a forum for a series of articles debating pain's meaning. According to a Dr. Gillies,

> I do not concern myself with definitions of pain. It is not the Whence nor the How of pain that is of practical interest, but the Wherefore—its meaning, intention, and purpose. . . . Pain never comes where it can serve no good purpose.

A Dr. Collins responded vehemently:

> Is this the grim comfort he would bring to a suffering woman tortured slowly to death by a sloughing *scirrhus* of the breast, or to a man, made almost inhuman and killed by inches by the slow yet sure ravages of a rodent ulcer?

As science and religion did battle in the nineteenth-century mind, the concept of pain was revolutionized. Pain was no longer seen as either a stepping-stone to spiritual enlightenment or as a punishment from God. Instead, for the first time it was viewed as a bodily function that could be removed—or at least diminished—by

Modern Religion and Pain

Recent studies show that patients with strong spirituality are able to manage their pain better without medication or with lower levels of medication. Research indicates spiritual beliefs have real health benefits:

- People with high levels of religious beliefs or spirituality have lower cortisol responses. Cortisol is a hormone the body releases in response to stress.
- Positive thinking produces nearly a 30 percent drop in perception of pain.
- Spirituality and the practice of religion have recently been associated with a slower progression of Alzheimer's disease.
- Those who regularly attend organized religious activities may live longer than those who don't. Regular participation lowers mortality rate by about 12 percent a year.
- People undergoing cardiac rehabilitation feel more confident and perceive greater improvements in their physical abilities if they have a strong faith.
- Increased levels of spirituality and religious faith may help substance abusers kick their habit.

medicine or surgery. God no longer held the keys to pain; doctors did.

By the twentieth century, various forms of painkillers had been developed and more were being researched. Pain had become something to be alleviated at all costs. It was not an experience filled with meaning; it was unnatural, unbearable, and doctors owed their patients a cure.

Modern Pain

In Norman Cousins' book *Anatomy of an Illness*, he writes, "Americans are the most pain-conscious people on the face of the earth." Cross-cultural studies of Americans,

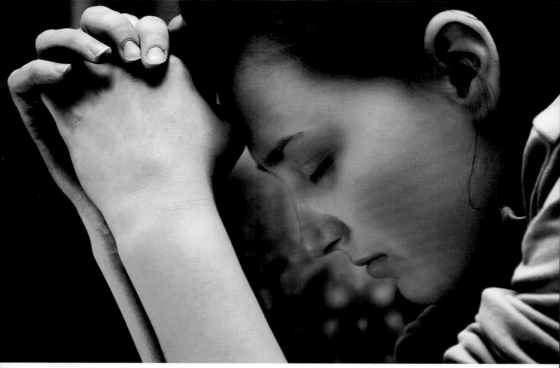

Scientific research indicates that spiritual practices increase a person's ability to cope with pain.

Japanese, and New Zealanders with lower back pain found that more Americans were seen for this disorder, took more medications for it, and were significantly more hindered from living out their everyday lives by their pain than were members of the other two groups. Another study found that white Americans with rheumatoid arthritis complained more often of pain than did Native Americans with the same disease. Stories from various native groups around the world report that childbirth in these cultures is associated with very little pain; meanwhile, in the Western world, women use a variety of medical interventions that allow them to escape the severe and nearly unbearable pain of childbirth.

In America, chronic pain can also entitle a person to disability payments; in other words, Americans see work and pain as mutually exclusive. Where earlier generations would have continued to work despite their pain (and

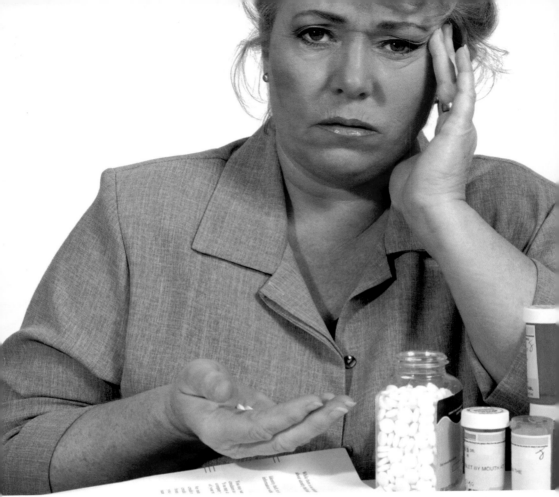

In today's world, most people expect to be able to take a pill to relieve their pain.

perhaps been distracted from their pain in the process), Americans have come to believe that pain is a condition that is insurmountable—and that ultimately, if they are forced to endure it, they deserve to be paid for it.

Pain and Pharmaceutical Companies

Pharmaceutical companies are major players in today's world. They help shape not only the medical world, but the financial and cultural worlds as well.

Prior to 1906, anybody with a recipe for a cure, a bit of charm, and the motivation to make some money could sell concoctions and call them medicine. To a large extent, the pharmaceutical industry was ruled by the profit motive, and salespeople peddled hopes rather than cures. It was in this atmosphere that the pharmaceutical industry had its start. Fortunately, the effectiveness of genuine drugs slowly became apparent, and in time those companies that made ineffective products failed. As more *potent* medicines became available and more money was spent on advertising them, expenditures on drugs rose dramatically.

In 1859, just prior to the American Civil War, sales of manufactured medicines reached about 3.5 million dollars per year. By 1904, sales of manufactured medicines had risen to almost 75 million dollars per year. Today, the North American pharmaceutical industry is huge, with

Drug Approval

Before a drug can be marketed in the United States, it must be officially approved by the Food and Drug Administration (FDA). Today's FDA is the primary consumer protection agency in the United States. Operating under the authority given it by the government, and guided by laws established throughout the twentieth century, the FDA has established a rigorous drug approval process that verifies the safety, effectiveness, and accuracy of labeling for any drug marketed in the United States.

While the United States has the FDA for the approval and regulation of drugs and medical devices, Canada has a similar organization called the Therapeutic Product Directorate (TPD). The TPD is a division of Health Canada, the Canadian government's department of health. The TPD regulates drugs, medical devices, disinfectants, and sanitizers with disinfectant claims. Some of the things that the TPD monitors are quality, effectiveness, and safety. Just as the FDA must approve new drugs in the United States, the TPD must approve new drugs in Canada before those drugs can enter the market.

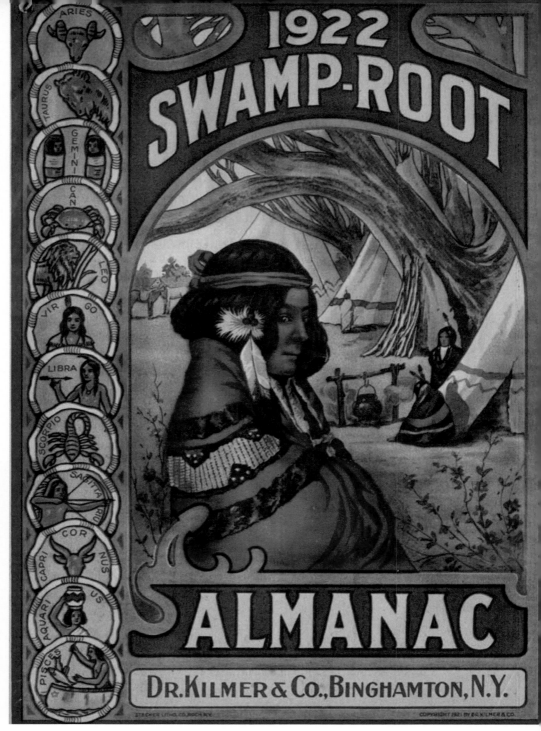

Early drug companies produced entire almanacs to advertise their products and lend credibility to their claims. Unfortunately, little if any scientific research supported these so-called medicines. Dr. Kilmer's Swamproot was one such popular medicine.

annual sales of prescription drugs topping 200 billion dollars in 2002.

Although the science behind drug development and the technology behind the manufacture of drugs have continued to progress throughout the history of the pharmaceutical industry, it was not until World War II that the pace of development truly leaped forward. World War II created a tremendous demand for new, more effective medical compounds, largely to treat injured and sick soldiers. Painkillers were just one of the many medicines wounded soldiers needed. After World War II, as industry and science turned their efforts away from wartime research and development and back toward more peaceful pursuits, the pharmaceutical industry entered a period of explosive growth and development that has continued to this day.

How Marketing Shapes Our Culture

Perhaps the most accurate and thorough explanation of marketing comes from the British Institute of Marketing, which defines marketing as "assessing and converting customer purchasing power into effective demand for a specific product." In other words, effective marketing is not simply the act of making consumers aware of a product. Rather, it is the act and process of making buyers feel as though they need that product.

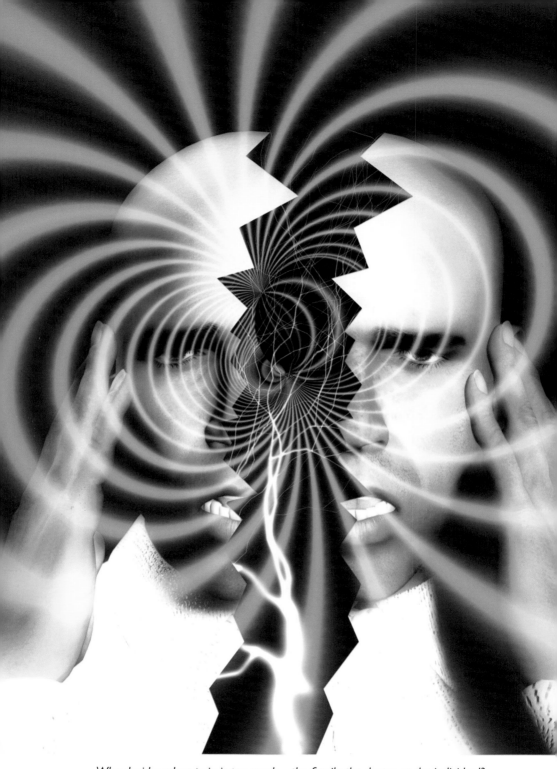

Who decides when pain is too much—the family, the doctor, or the individual?

30 Chapter 2—The History of Pain

Nowhere is the conversion of buying power into demand more readily visible than in the market for drugs. One way that drug companies create a demand for particular drugs is by making consumers more aware of the condition the drug treats. By "teaching" consumers about depression, pharmaceutical companies created a greater market for these medications—and by educating consumers about pain management, they did the same thing for painkillers.

In 1997, the U.S. Food and Drug Administration (FDA) loosened restrictions against direct-to-consumer advertising—commonly abbreviated DTC advertising—of prescription medicines. Before that, most advertisements for prescription drugs could not link the name of a drug to the conditions it treated. In other words, most advertisements mentioned either the drug name or the condition it treated, but not both. While this approach could help motivate more people to seek medical advice on a condition they might be suffering, it clearly is not very useful for companies trying to get people to use their product for that condition. In general then, pharmaceutical companies only advertised to physicians and other medical professionals through specialized medical and

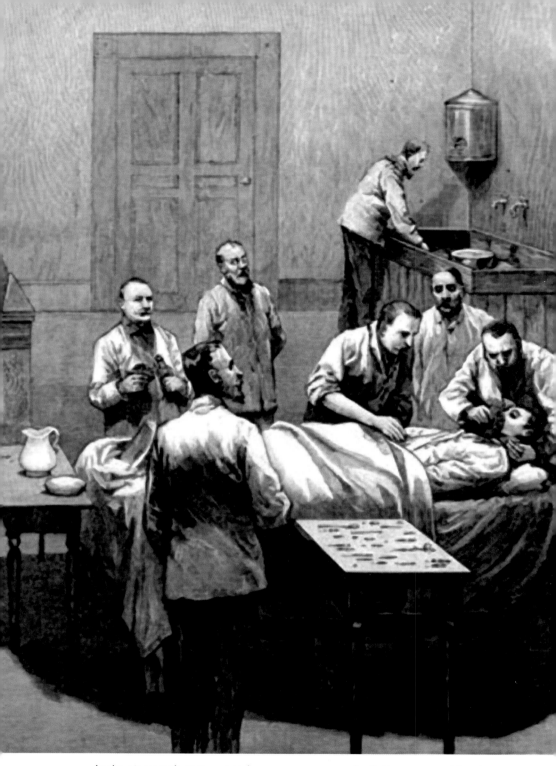

In the nineteenth century, painless surgery as a result of ether was considered a miracle of modern science.

scientific journals, and through the visits of pharmaceutical salespeople.

In Canada and most other countries in the world, DTC advertising is still illegal. However, a huge number of stations that broadcast on Canadian television and radio originate in the United States and carry American advertising. In addition, many magazines and newspapers come to Canada from the United States. Internet advertising too has grown, and American companies have taken full advantage of its power to reach many people. Despite the Canadian government's stance against DTC advertising, nearly as much advertising for painkillers and other prescription drugs bombards Canadians as it does Americans.

There is little *consensus* as to whether this is a good thing, but there can be little doubt that the rise of DTC advertising in the United States has had a significant impact on the way pharmaceutical companies do business. In the process, they have greater power to shape the way Americans think—including their perceptions of pain and pain management.

With the use of ether as an anesthetic in the late nineteenth century, physicians thought pain would be virtually eliminated. Obviously, that did not prove to be the case. The ongoing search for total pain relief has led to the development of a multitude of painkillers. When the availability of these painkillers combined with Western culture, the results were both positive and negative.

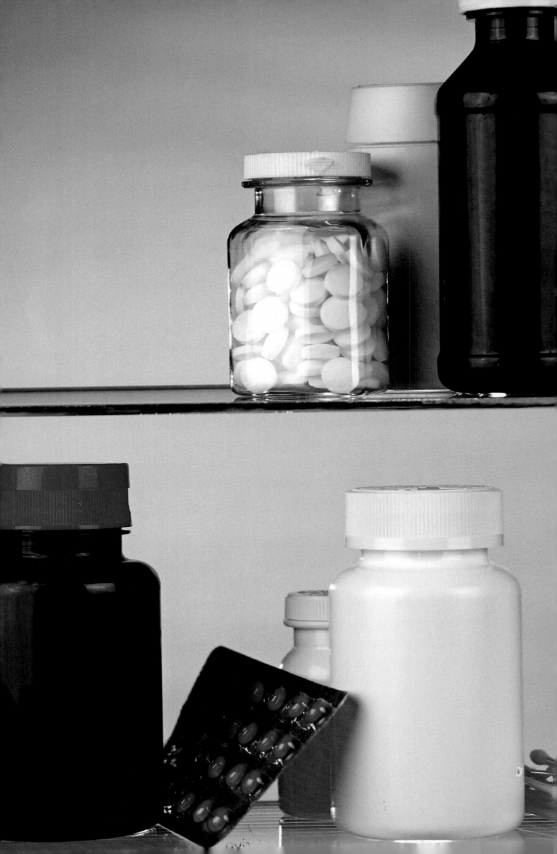

3 The Painkillers

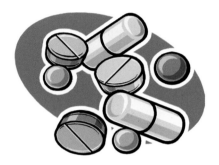

Most people have acetaminophen, ibuprofen, or naproxen in their medicine cabinet, more commonly known as Tylenol®, Advil®, and Aleve®. Along with aspirin (acetylsalicylic acid), they are the basic pain relievers available over the counter. Though they vary in potency, indications, and **contraindications**, they are all part of the drug classification analgesics. An analgesic is a type of medication that eases pain but does not cause unconsciousness; analgesics treat the pain, not the source of the injury or disease causing the pain. There are three categories of analgesics: opioids, nonopioids, and combined analgesics.

Opioids

Opioids have been used for pleasure and to relieve pain for millennia. The pleasure-giving properties of the opium poppy, the original source of opium, was known as far back as 3400 BCE, when the Sumerians called the flower the "joy plant." Opioid use spread from Egypt to Greece by 1300 BCE. The physician and *alchemist* Paracelsus introduced opium to Europeans in 1527 as a medical treatment. During the late 1800s, opioid abuse spread with the development of the hypodermic needle, which allowed the user to achieve a quicker effect.

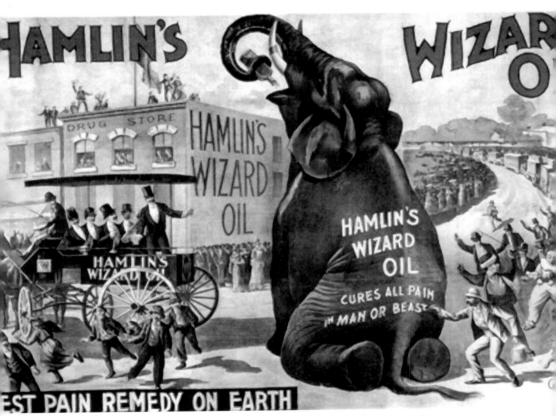

Hamlin's Wizard Oil was an effective pain reliever—thanks to opium, its main ingredient.

36   Chapter 3—The Painkillers

If you had a cough in the eighteenth century, your doctor might have suggested you dose yourself with the following medication: *a teacupful of opium syrup three or four times a day.* Or, if you suffered from headaches, he would have been likely to prescribe an opium powder for you to take. These medicines were all perfectly legal in the 1700s.

Opium was marketed under a variety of labels such as these:

- Ayer's Cherry Pectoral,
- Mrs. Winslow's Soothing Syrup,
- McMunn's Elixer,
- Godfrey's Cordial,
- Hamlin's Wizard Oil,
- Scott's Emulsion
- Dover's Powder.

These remedies were advertised as "painkillers," "cough mixtures," "soothing syrups," and "women's

Dating Systems and Their Meaning

You might be accustomed to seeing dates expressed with the abbreviations BC or AD, as in the year 1000 BC or the year AD 1900. For centuries, this dating system has been the most common in the Western world. However, since BC and AD are based on Christianity (BC stands for Before Christ and AD stands for anno *Domini*, Latin for "in the year of our Lord"), many people now prefer to use abbreviations that people from all religions can be comfortable using. The abbreviations BCE (meaning Before Common Era) and CE (meaning Common Era) mark time in the same way (for example, 1000 BC is the same year as 1000 BCE, and AD 1900 is the same year as 1900 CE), but BCE and CE do not have the same religious overtones as BC and AD.

friends." They were used to treat everyone from rheumatic grandparents to teething babies. The medicine may have soothed the patients' pain, but as a result many people, including babies, suffered addiction, withdrawal pains, and even death. And yet the medicine was thought to cure diarrhea, colds, cholera, fever, cancer—and even baldness and athlete's foot!

Opioids are still considered one of the most highly effective and well tolerated of the analgesics. Also called prescription narcotics, opioids are among the most commonly prescribed painkillers today. Opioids are derived from opium, or can be any narcotic with opiate-like effects. Among the most common opioids are morphine, codeine, and diphenoxylate. Doctors prescribe these medications to treat moderate to severe pain and to control the pain of postsurgical patients. Codeine and diphenoxylate can also be used to treat diarrhea and severe and chronic coughs. Morphine can be processed to produce the more rapid-acting opioid, heroin, which is sought after by abusers and still sold in the United Kingdom for pain relief. Methadone is yet

Brand Name vs. Generic Name

Talking about medications can be confusing because every drug has at least two names: its "generic name" and the "brand name" that the pharmaceutical company uses to market the drug. Generic names are based on the drug's chemical structure, while drug companies use brand names in order to inspire public recognition and loyalty for their products.

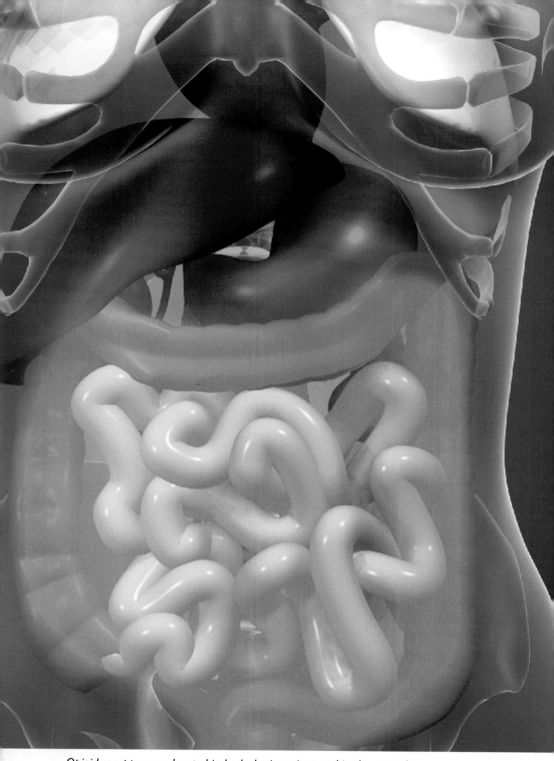

Opioid receptors are located in both the intestines and in the central nervous system.

The National Institute on Drug Abuse lists some of the uses and consequences of opioids in its 2005 report:

Use and Consequences of Opioids
Opioids
- Oxycodone
- Propoxyphene
- Hydrocodone
- Hydromorphone
- Meperidine
- Diphenoxylate
- Morphine
- Codeine
- Fentanyl
- Methadone

Generally prescribed for
- postsurgical pain relief
- management of acute or chronic pain
- relief of cough and diarrhea

Effects of short-term use
- alleviates pain
- drowsiness
- constipation
- depressed respiration (depending on dose)

Effect of long-term use
- potential for physical dependence and addiction

Possible negative effects
- severe respiratory depression or death following a large single dose

Should not be used with
other substances that cause central nervous system depression, including:
- alcohol
- antihistamines
- barbiturates
- benzodiazepines
- general anesthetics

(*Source:* From *National Institute on Drug Abuse Research Report,* August 2005)

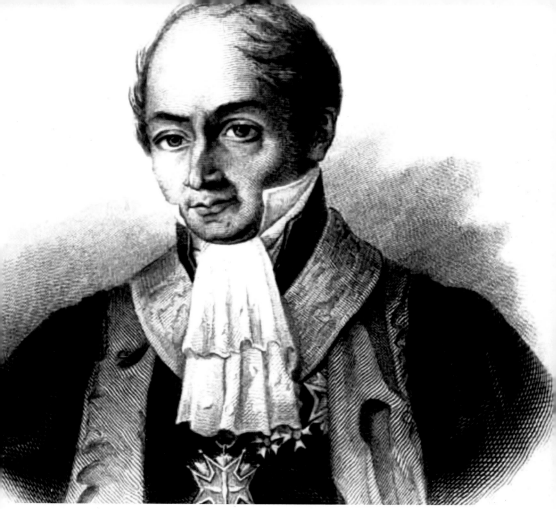

Morphine was discovered by Friedrich Sertürner, a German pharmacist, early in the nineteenth century.

another opioid that provides effective pain relief when given orally and is also used as a relatively safe substitute for heroin during addiction treatment.

How Opioids Work

Receptors, proteins located on cell membranes or within the **cytoplasm**, bind to a specific molecule. This molecule is called a ligand, and the receptors spark the cells' response to that specific molecule. This response causes a physiological change. In the case of painkillers such as morphine, codeine, and diphenoxylate, the opioids attach themselves to an opioid receptor located in the CNS and **gastrointestinal** tract. When a drug such as Percocet® attaches to an opioid receptor, it blocks the brain's perception of pain. Some of the potential side effects of opioid use are drowsiness, nausea, constipation, and respiratory problems. Because the drug affects the region of the brain associated with pleasure sensations, **euphoria** can also result. This feeling is intensified if the drug is abused or taken in a nonrecommended form, such as snorting or injecting OxyContin®, a brand-name of a long-acting form of oxycodone.

When taken as directed by a medical professional, opioids are a safe way to manage pain in the short term. They have not been found to be addictive when taken properly. Like all other drugs, opioids should not be combined with another medication—over the counter or prescription—except under the supervision of a health-care professional. Life-threatening respiratory distress can be caused when they are used with alcohol, antihistamines, barbiturates, or benzodiazepines.

Morphine

Morphine is the primary active ingredient in opium. The drug was isolated in 1804 by the German pharmacist Friedrich Sertürner. The word "morphine" comes from Morpheus, the Greek god of dreams.

Like other opiates, the use of morphine spread with the introduction of the hypodermic needle in the mid-nineteenth century. The drug was used as a cure for opium and alcohol addiction. It's effectiveness as a pain reliever was soon apparent, and its use skyrocketed during the Civil War when it was used to treat wounds. According to some researchers, so many military personnel became addicted to it that opioid dependence was called the "soldier's disease." Doctors and patients both came to rely on the instant relief supplied by morphine. In fact, it was used so often that the 1897 edition of the Sears Roebuck catalog offered a hypodermic kit—a syringe, two needles, two vials, and a handy carrying case for one's personal supply of morphine. The entire kit cost $1.50.

In 1874, heroin (diacetylmorphine) was first *synthesized* in Germany. The word "heroin" is derived from the German word *heroisch*, which means heroic. At first, heroin was considered a safe substitute for morphine. It took many years before the dangerous addictive qualities of heroin were discovered. Dr. Heinrich Dreser of the Bayer Company, makers of the aspirin, introduced heroin as a cough suppressant and pain reliever in 1898.

Today, morphine is generally given by an injection or through an IV drip; only rarely is it given as a liquid or in pill form. It is also available in autoinjectors, and reportedly, some military forces provide these injectors to their units. The drug acts directly on the CNS to relieve pain and is highly effective. It is marketed under such names as Avinza®, Kadian®, and Roxanol®.

Potential side effects of the drug include:

- impairment of mental performance
- euphoria
- drowsiness
- lethargy
- blurred vision
- decreased appetite
- inhibition of the cough reflex
- constipation

Morphine is highly addictive, and prolonged use builds up tolerance in the user. Someone who has used morphine for more than five to seven days should not stop taking it at once. To do so may cause serious withdrawal symptoms. Doctors will gradually reduce the dosage so that withdrawal symptoms are minimized. If the dose reduction is done too rapidly, the patient may experience the flu-like symptoms of opioid withdrawal. With proper medical monitoring, few patients develop an addiction.

Codeine

Codeine (methylmorphine) is the most widely used, naturally occurring narcotic being used in medical treat-

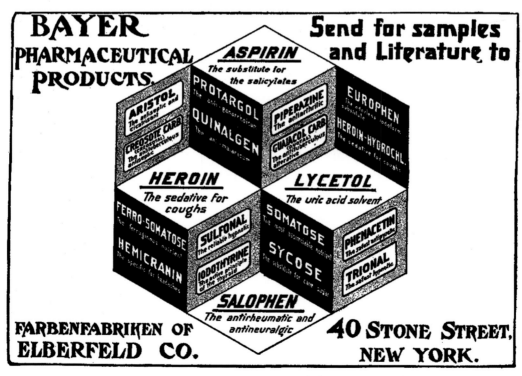

An early Bayer advertisement introduced several of its products, including aspirin and heroin.

ment in the world today. An **alkaloid**, codeine is found in opium. However, most codeine in use in the United States today is synthesized from morphine and combined with other pain relievers.

Today, the primary use of codeine is for the relief of moderate pain and for cough suppression. It is usually taken orally, and is sometimes combined with acetaminophen or ibuprofen. Although it has less severe side effects than morphine, it is not side effect free. Potential side effects include:

- itching
- nausea and vomiting
- drowsiness
- dry mouth
- urinary retention
- constipation

Like morphine, users should not suddenly stop taking the medication. A physician-directed tapering of the dosage will help keep withdrawal symptoms to a minimum.

Oxycodone

Oxycodone is one of the strongest pain control medications that can be taken orally. It is synthesized from thebaine, a poisonous alkaloid component of opium that causes convulsions similar to those caused by **strychnine**. It is combined with acetaminophen and sold as Percocet, one of the most often prescribed medications for post-surgical pain. The acetaminophen helps relatively small doses of oxycodone effectively treat pain, but people that use too much for too long can develop liver disease, due to the acetaminophen. Combined with aspirin, it is

Common Nonopioids

Etodolac
Fenoprofen
Ketoprofen
Mefenamic Acid
Piroxicam

Common NSAIDs

aspirin
diclofenac
ibuprofen
naproxen

marketed as Percodan. The aspirin, like acetaminophen, helps smaller doses of oxycodone reduce pain, but some people develop stomach upset due to the combination. A sustained release form, OxyContin, has brought pain relief to many who had suffered for years. It has the advantage of not including acetaminophen or aspirin and could be given at higher doses to relieve severe chronic pain. It has also brought much controversy and abuse to a new group of people (see chapter 5).

Doctors generally prescribe oxycodone for moderate to severe pain and for no more than several weeks. When taken as directed, it has been found to provide effective pain management with moderate side effects. These can include:

- nausea
- constipation
- lightheadedness
- rash
- dizziness
- emotional mood disorders

If treatment extends for several months, tolerance and dependence may occur, requiring larger doses to get the same effect. According to the Drug Enforcement Agency (DEA), psychological addiction brought on by proper medical use is rare. However, there are outstanding lawsuits that argue to the contrary.

Other Prescription Painkillers

Weak or "Partial" Morphine-Like Opioids

Some opioids only partially produce morphine-like effects. These can be used with less risk of addiction or lethal overdose.

One is called buprenorphine. In small does it is effective for pain relief, but it is not as strong as morphine. In higher doses it can be used to treat addiction to heroin and other opioids by providing a partial substitute. This drug is replacing methadone in heroin addiction treatment because of its safety advantages, a fact that has been recognized by both Congress and the U.S. Food and Drug Administration. Laws have been passed allowing people

The History of Aspirin

Hippocrates, the father of modern medicine who lived sometime between 460 and 377 BCE, left historical records of a powder made from the bark and leaves of the willow tree, which he used to relieve headaches and other pains. Native Americans also recognized the medical properties of the willow tree; they chewed the willow's leaves and inner bark or boiled a tea made from them to relieve fever or other minor pain like toothaches, headaches, or arthritis. By 1829, scientists discovered that it was the compound called salicin in willow plants that gave you the pain relief. Aspirin was patented on March 6, 1889, by a German company called Bayer. The folks at Bayer came up with the name aspirin, using the "A" in acetyl chloride (the chemical compound contained in salicin), the "spir" in spiraea ulmaria (the genus of plant containing this compound) and "in," which was a then familiar name ending for medicines. Aspirin was first sold as a powder, but in 1915, the first aspirin tablets were made.

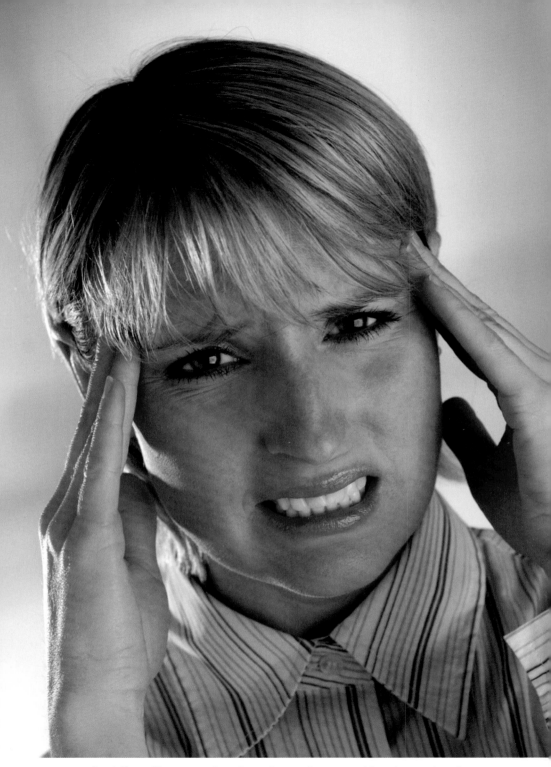

Painkillers offer genuine benefits to human beings, enabling them to live their lives free from discomfort and pain.

to be treated for addiction with burprenorphine outside of regular doctors' offices.

Tremadol is another example of a drug that is chemically related to opioids. Many of its morphine-like effects, however, are so weak that its risk of addiction is very low. A prescription is needed to purchase this drug, but is not regulated as stringently as morphine-like opioids.

Opioid Antagonists

Still another category of opioids are the drugs that block the effects of morphine-like opioids. These are called antagonists. Naloxone is a short-acting example of one of these drugs that is given by injection. Naltrexone lasts a few days and can be given orally. Both drugs are used in hospitals to help doctors in case they gave too much of a morphine-like opioid. They are also used to reverse the effects of heroin overdose. When given by injection, they act so rapidly that a person near death from opioid overdose may open her eyes, sit up, and begin talking less than a minute after the injection. Opioid-addicted people can be treated with naltrexone because in they take a morphine-like opioid while on naltrexone, they will experience either no effect of even withdrawal.

Nonopioids

Although opioids are by far the most-prescribed and most-abused painkillers, less severe pain may be treated with nonopioids, also called non-narcotics. They are often used to treat headaches, toothaches, muscle and joint pains, and menstrual cramps. Though many of these medications can be purchased over the counter, higher dosages are usually available only with a prescription.

Some nonopioids also act as anti-inflammatories. Injuries such as sprains or chronic conditions like arthritis can cause body tissues to release chemicals called prosta-glandins. The prostaglandins can cause the area around the injury to swell and redden, causing pain. Anti-inflammatories block swelling, thereby easing pain. Some anti-inflammatories use steroids, while others do not. Anti-inflammatory nonopioids do not contain steroids and are called nonsteroidal anti-inflammatory drugs (NSAIDs).

NSAIDs can take away pain, or if it is more severe, "take the edge off" the pain, lessening the need to take stronger medications such as codeine or morphine. Addiction is not a problem with NSAIDs and nonopioids. They are not, however, without potential side effects. They can hinder blood clotting, and with prolonged use, can cause stomach bleeding. Nausea and indigestion are also possible. Use of NSAIDs and nonopioids may also lead to kidney disorders, especially if alcohol is consumed on a regular basis. There have also been reports of slow healing of bones in people taking NSAIDs.

Combined Analgesics

The third category of painkillers is combined analgesics. These drugs combine a mild nonopioid drug (such as aspirin) with a small amount of an opioid in a single pill. One of the most common combinations is Tylenol with codeine. These medications are designed for those whose pain is not being relieved by nonopioids alone, and for whom standard dosages of an opioid are contraindicated. Although most combined analgesics are available only with a prescription, some, with a smaller dose of the opioid, are available over the counter.

The very existence of painkillers is linked to North Americans' ideas about pain. If pain is a completely bad thing, then we should do all that we can to avoid it—and we look to medicine to offer us relief. Unfortunately, these medications can also be abused.

Clearly, painkillers are not necessarily bad things; taken as prescribed or recommended by a physician, these medications can alleviate pain, allowing individuals to lead a life of quality. However, like many things that have started out with the best of intentions, prescription medications have become drugs of choice for some abusers.

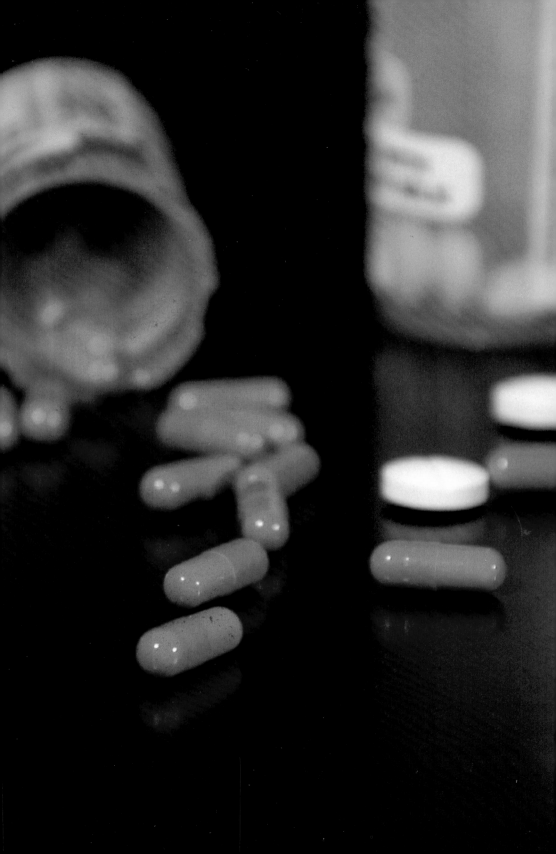

The Abuse of Prescription Painkillers

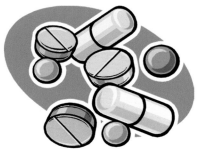

The nonmedical use of prescription drugs, including painkillers, has increased dramatically in the past few years. (The National Survey on Drug Use and Health, NSDUH) defines nonmedical use as occurring when an individual takes prescription medications that were not prescribed for her, or takes the medication only for the feeling—the "high"—that results from taking it.) According to the Drug Abuse Warning Network, which monitors cases of illicit drug admissions to hospital emergency rooms, opioid pain relievers accounted for 119,000 emergency room visits in 2002.

The NSDUH also asked survey respondents to evaluate symptoms of dependence on or abuse of painkillers. Criteria from the *Diagnostic and Statistical Manual of*

Mental Disorders, Fourth Edition (DSM-IV) were used to assess dependence and abuse. These symptoms included:

- withdrawal
- tolerance
- use in dangerous situations
- trouble with the law
- interference in major obligations at work, school, or home during the previous year

Who Is Abusing Prescription Pain Relievers?

Although overall drug use among teenagers is down (between 1998 and 2004, the use of marijuana, for example, decreased 42 percent), the nonmedical use of prescription medications has increased. This trend toward the nonmedical use of prescription medications has caused some to refer to this generation of teenagers as "Generation Rx." In 2005, Steve Pasierb, president and chief execu-

Drugs Used Most Nonmedically

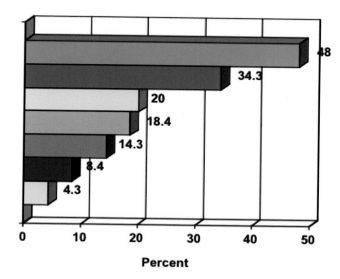

	Percent
Vicodin, Lortab, or Lorcet	48
Darvocet, Darvon, or Tylenol with Codeine	34.3
Percocet, Percodan, or Tylox	20
Hydrocodone	18.4
Codeine	14.3
OxyContin	8.4
Morphine	4.3

Source: U.S. Substance Abuse and Mental Health Services Administration

tive officer of the Partnership for a Drug-Free America, is quoted in the *Washington Times* as saying that this trend has been "one of the most significant developments in substance abuse trends in recent memory." According to its 2004 survey of teen drug abuse, the Partnership for a Drug-Free America also found that one in five teens has abused Vicodin, and one in ten has used OcyContin, both for nonmedical purposes. Thirty-seven percent of respondents indicated that they have close friends who have used prescription painkillers nonmedically. The trend continued in the Partnership for a Drug-Free

According to Canadian statistics, the nonmedical use of opioid painkillers in Canada has increased at such a staggering rate since the late 1990s, that these users outnumber street heroin users in some treatment populations. Because of the rampant abuse of these drugs, officials are finding it difficult to curtail their illegal use while making certain that they remain available for those who truly need them.

Street Names for Opioids

- ac/dc
- baby blues
- coties
- demmies
- dillies
- hillbilly heroin
- o.c.
- oxy
- oxycotton
- percs
- vics

America's 2005 survey. According to the Web site www. drugfree.org, the use of prescription and over-the-counter medications has become "entrenched in today's teen population."

Most teenage survey participants indicated that they used prescription medication as their drug of choice because it was easily obtainable; after all, prescription medications can be found in the medicine cabinets in many homes. A study conducted by the National Institute on Drug Abuse (NIDA) in 2004 found that, in some areas, teens would gather up old prescription medications, get together with other teens at "pharming parties," and trade for other prescription drugs. At some parties, teens bring whatever prescription drugs they find in their medicine cabinets, throw them all into a bowl and pass it around, taking whatever they want; this is the "salad bowl." There are also many Internet sites offering prescription drugs such as OxyContin and Vicodin, some advertising that a prescription is not needed. A Google search on July 5, 2006, for "no prescription needed OxyContin" brought up almost two million hits. Although businesses may ad-

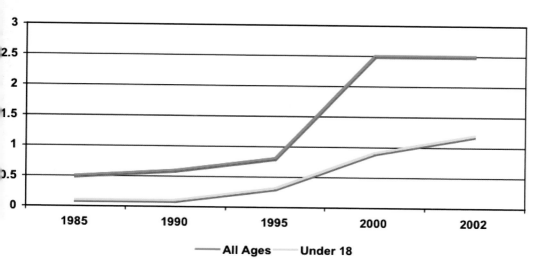

Millions of Persons Who First Used Pain Relievers Nonmedically in the United States 1985–2002

All Ages — Under 18

Source: U.S. Substance Abuse and Mental Health Services Administration

vertise that prescriptions are not necessary, it is illegal to purchase such **controlled substances** without one.

Another reason teens are turning to prescription medications, including painkillers, is that they consider them to be safer than street drugs; a little less than 50 percent of those surveyed did not see a major risk in taking prescription medications. After all, these medications were prescribed by a physician or other health-care professional

Good News

According to a 2004 NIDA study, the number of U.S. students in grades 8, 10, and 12 who admitted to using drugs during the previous thirty days dropped 17 percent from 2001.

Bad News

The same study reported that between 2002 and 2004, the use of OxyContin increased significantly in teens.

permitted by law to do so. If the medications were available for dispensing, they had to have been approved by the Food and Drug Administration in the United States or the Therapeutic Product Directorate in Canada. What some teens fail to realize, is that the medications are approved for use for a specific purpose (and that purpose is *not* getting high) and under the direction of a health-care professional. Adding to this possible false sense of security, nearly one-third of the respondents thought they could not become addicted to prescription painkillers, unlike most street drugs. Advertising on television and in other media have made the teenage abuser well educated about the brand names of and effects caused by many of these prescription medications.

Gender and race were also factors in the nonmedical use of prescription painkillers according to the previously cited NSDUH study. In its 2002 survey, it was found that males were more likely than females to have used prescription painkillers nonmedically at some point during

Troubling Trends

- Pharming—kids "getting high" abusing prescription or over-the-counter drugs.
- It has never been easier to get high; Internet accessibility and loose e-commerce enforcement further enable easy acquisition.
- Parents do not understand the behavior of intentionally abusing medicine to get high.
- Three out of five parents report discussing marijuana "a lot" with their children, but only one-third of parents report discussing the risks of using prescription medicines or nonprescription cold or cough medicine to get high.

(Source: From "Key Findings on Teen Drug Trends (PATS 2005)," www.drug-free.org.)

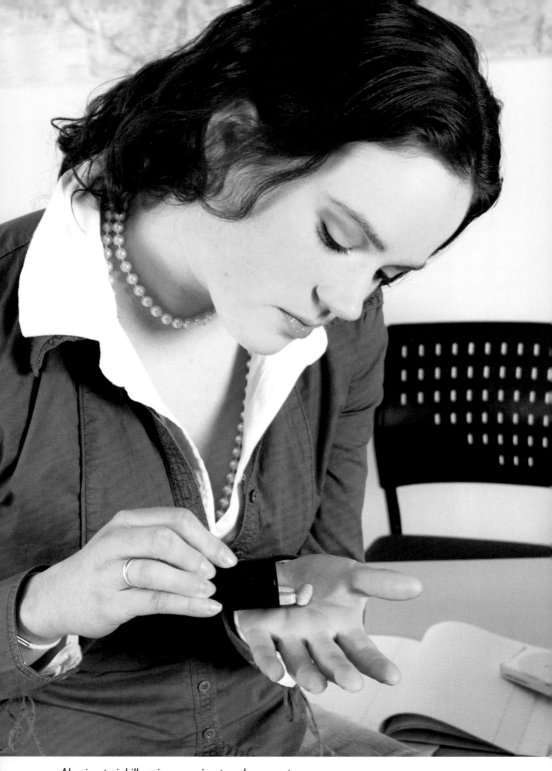

Abusing painkillers is a growing trend among teens.

their lifetime, 14.3 percent to 11.0 percent, respectively. Whites (13.6 percent) were more likely to have done so, followed by Hispanics (11.0 percent), blacks (9.7 percent), and Asians (7.0 percent).

Residents of small metropolitan areas were more likely to have used prescription painkillers nonmedically at any point during their lifetime (13.7 percent) than people who lived in large metropolitan areas (12.4 percent) or nonmetropolitan areas (11.2 percent).

Statistics for dependence during the past twelve months differ from those reflecting nonmedical use of prescription painkillers over one's lifetime. There is almost no difference between the percentage of males and females who reported a dependence on prescription painkillers during the previous twelve months (0.7 percent and 0.6 percent, respectively). During the past year, Hispanics are the most likely group to have developed a dependency (0.9 percent). They are followed by whites (0.7 percent), blacks (0.4 percent), and Asians (0.1 percent). People in small metropolitan areas are almost twice as likely to have been dependent on prescription painkillers than those living in rural and large metropolitan areas (0.9 percent, compared with 0.5 percent for both nonmetropolitan and large metropolitan areas).

How Addiction Develops

Like many other people, Sylvia's doctor put her on Vicodin because she suffered from chronic migraines. The pills worked effectively. They took away her headaches and allowed her to live her life. But, like other narcotics, Vicodin lost its effectiveness over time. Sylvia began to increase her

NSDUH-Reported Prescription Painkillers of Choice

In 2002, the most prevalent prescription painkillers used nonmedically by individuals age twelve and over were:

Darvocet, Darvon, or Tylenol with Codeine	18.9 percent
Vicodin, Lortab, of Lorcet	13.1 percent
Percocet, Percodan, or Tylox	9.7 percent

(Source: The NSDUH Report, May 21, 2004.)

dosage. She had built up a tolerance to the medication. She was physically dependent on Vicodin.

Fearing that her doctor would stop prescribing the medication if she told him that she had increased the dosage, she kept it a secret. She did not believe that she would be able to function without the pills. She began to change the numbers on the prescriptions so that she would get more pills, with more refills.

Over the next two years, she went from a physical dependence to a physical and psychological addiction. She had to continue to take this drug in increasing dosages in order to feel "normal." She went from taking the medication as prescribed to a drug habit of 30 pills a day. She started to "*doctor shop*" in order to obtain several prescriptions at a time. . . . She switched pharmacies in different neighborhoods so that no one would become suspicious.

She could not use her insurance since she was buying several prescriptions of Vicodin at one time. She used different names at each pharmacy. She spent hundreds of dollars a month. She kept a careful record of who she was at every one. As her

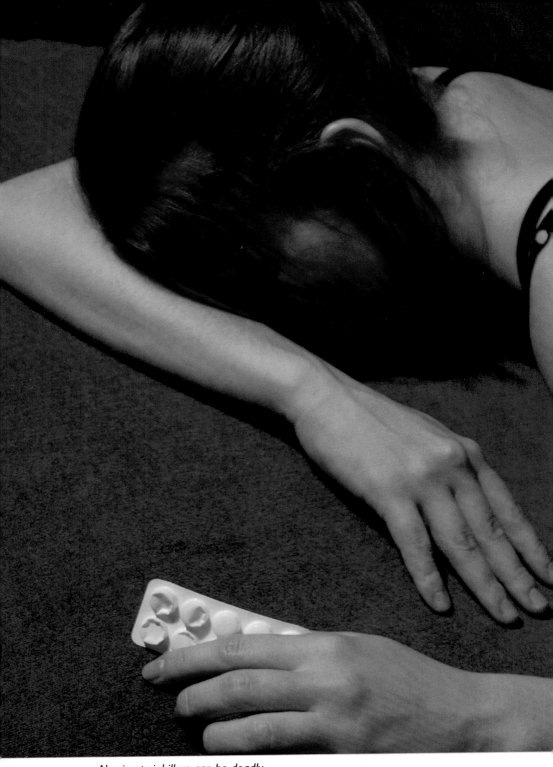

Abusing painkillers can be deadly.

habit increased, she had to find new ways of getting pills. She stole a prescription pad from one of her doctors and began to forge her own prescriptions. One day, she made the mistake of writing a date on the forged prescription that happened to be a Sunday. The pharmacist became suspicious and confronted her about it. She quickly left the store. He called the police.

By the time the police raided her house, she had hundreds of pills hidden in the bathroom, the kitchen, and bedroom. The police thought she was selling them. They had no idea that the amount she had wouldn't even last her two weeks. (*Source:* www.prescription-drug-abuse.org.)

From a picnic-style table in a Perry County [Kentucky] jail, Donna Marie Couch tells the story of her Oxy [OxyContin] addiction. The 21-year-old has been doing drugs since she was 12.

"The first time," she says, "I snorted it at my house. When I done it, it relaxed me. It made me nod out. I liked them a lot."

That was three years ago. She used the drug nearly every day until she was arrested for breaking into a house.

Today, she's been behind bars for five months, part of a six-month sentence for the crime.

"I was just high," she says. "I didn't know what I was doing."

Before her incarceration, Ms. Couch did everything she could to get the drug. Her entire paycheck from a part-time job at Captain D's went to buy Oxy. She even did the drug alone so she wouldn't have to share.

Anyone Can Become Addicted

He's revered by millions of radio listeners called "Dittoheads." He's a best-selling author. He's addicted to prescription painkillers. He's conservative radio talk-show host Rush Limbaugh.

In 2003, his housekeeper confessed to Florida law enforcement authorities that she had bought OxyContin for Limbaugh. And she had the goods to back up her claims. According to a story in Newsweek magazine, she turned over ledgers and e-mails showing that Limbaugh had bought 30,000 prescription painkillers, including OxyContin and Lorcet.

Limbaugh admitted his abuse, saying he'd started taking pills for back pain. He voluntarily entered a thirty-day rehabilitation program and later cut a deal with the district attorney, allowing him to receive *probation* rather than incarceration. Apparently he forgot what he had once said on air about drug abusers: "'Too many whites are getting away with drug use. The answer is to . . . find the ones who are getting away with it, convict them, and send them up the river.'"

"I didn't care at the time," she says. "That's all I wanted. You really don't know that you're in that bad of shape."

When police busted her, they brought her in with a 300-milligram-a-day habit, enough to treat some chronic pain sufferers for five days. She weighed only 96 pounds. Her addiction had fractured her relationship with her mother and father. Her health deteriorated.

She vows that when she gets out next month she'll kick the habit, maybe even go to school in Alabama.

"It was crazy the things I was doing," she says. "(But) if you don't start, you don't have to stop."

(*Source: The Cincinnati Enquirer*, February 25, 2001.)

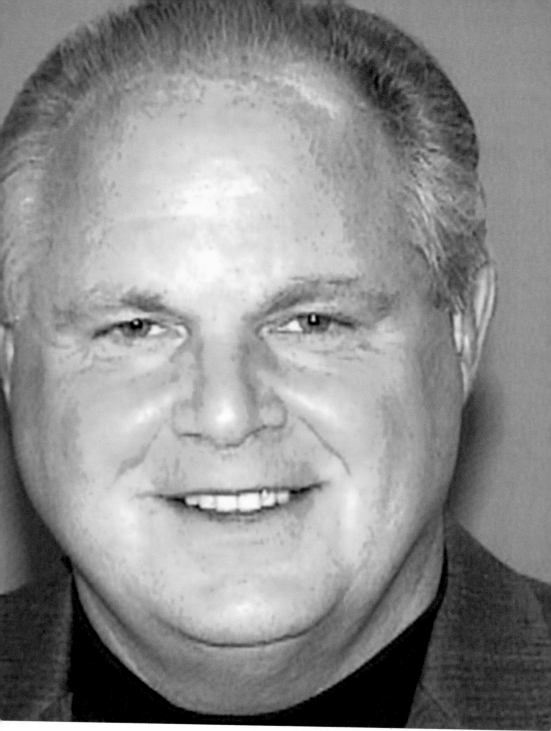

In April 2006, Rush Limbaugh was again in trouble over painkillers. He surrendered to the Palm Beach County Sheriff's Office after being charged with doctor shopping. According to investigators, Limbaugh bounced from doctors in a bid to secure multiple prescriptions for powerful painkillers like OxyContin.

Painkillers—Prescription Dependency 65

These stories tell how two users came to be addicted to prescription pain medications. Though they came to addiction in different ways, the result was the same: an illness that affected every part of their lives.

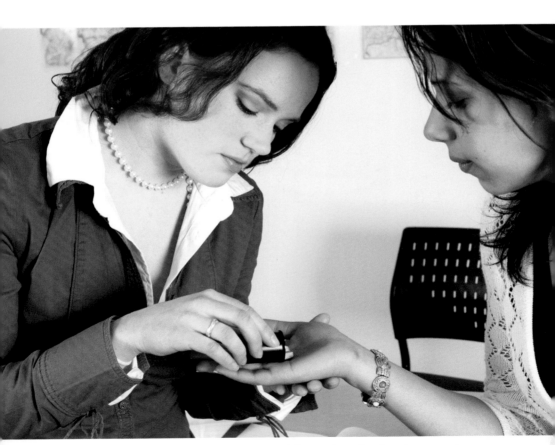

When friends share prescription painkillers with each other, they may also share addictions.

Having a drug dependency and being addicted to a drug are not the same things. After taking some medications for a period of time, the body may build up a tolerance toward the drug, and the person must take more of the medication to achieve the same effect. When someone stops taking the drug, she experiences withdrawal symptoms because her body has become dependent on the medication. By following the instructions of the health-care professional, dependence can be easily treated and withdrawal symptoms minimized and possibly eliminated with proper dosage adjustments.

Sometimes the need for the drug is more than physical. If an individual must take the drug to satisfy emotional and psychological needs, he is addicted. The person addicted to the drug has a *compulsive* need to use the medication for nonmedical purposes; the drug is taken because of its mood-altering effects, not to relieve pain. His behavior can become erratic and include stealing drugs

Abuse—or Misuse?

Abuse and misuse are two different things; unfortunately, both can lead to addiction.

Misuse:

Patients may forget or not understand their prescription's directions. They may start making their own decisions, perhaps upping the dose in hopes of getting better faster.

Abuse:

People may use prescription drugs for nonmedical reasons. Prescription drug abusers may obtain such drugs illegally and use them to get high, fight stress, or boost energy.

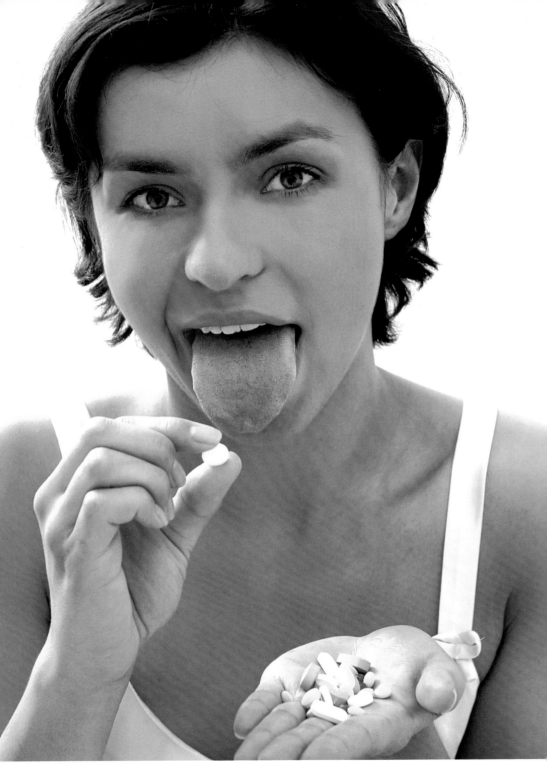

Sometimes addiction begins with a legitimate medical prescription.

from friends and family members and selling and buying drugs on the street. The addicted person may begin to lie, obsessively count the pills, steal prescription pads, forge doctors' signatures, and "doctor shop." He may return to his health-care provider and tell her that he "lost" his medication, that it fell into the toilet, or even that his dog ate it—all with the goal of getting more of the drug.

Although in Donna's case the prescription painkiller was just another substance in her drug-taking experience, Sylvia's involvement with prescription painkillers began with a legitimate medical prescription; she suffered from migraines, and Vicodin is an accepted medication for the condition. Her problem with Vicodin began when she increased her dosage of the medication, rather than explain to her health-care professional her concern that the medication was no longer working. With proper medical supervision, her dosage could have been adjusted to treat her migraines effectively. The doctor could have suggested other pain management techniques as well. But Sylvia's drug dependence turned into a true addiction, though not everyone who becomes dependent on a painkiller or other medication will proceed to develop an addiction.

Sylvia's case represents a major problem in pain management. Many people who have medical reasons for taking painkillers hesitate to do so in fear of becoming addicted to the drug. According to the Chronic Pain **Advocacy** League, the number of people who do so is small. Most people take the medication for short periods of time, usually from just a few days to a month. For those with chronic pain, the risk of addiction is greater but still small. According to Karen Miotto, a psychiatrist specializing in addiction and cited on www.medicinenet.com,

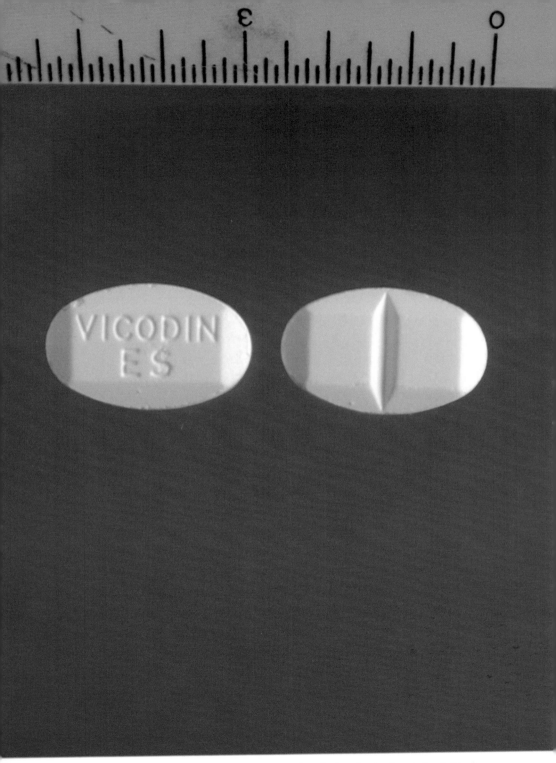

Vicodin is often prescribed for migraine headaches; it also has potential to be abused.

only an estimated 3 percent to 16 percent of people being treated with opioids for chronic pain become addicted. She hypothesizes that precipitating factors indicating the possibility of addiction include a personal or family history of addiction, or being under a great deal of stress. Research conducted by James Zacny, a professor in the department of anesthesia and critical care at the University of Chicago and cited on www.medicinenet.com, found that people who experienced a more positive effect from the drug—a high—may be more likely to develop an addiction.

Prescription painkillers have brought relief, and a significant improvement to the quality of life of many people. The *efficacy* of one such painkiller, however, has also made it one of the most infamous ones of our time.

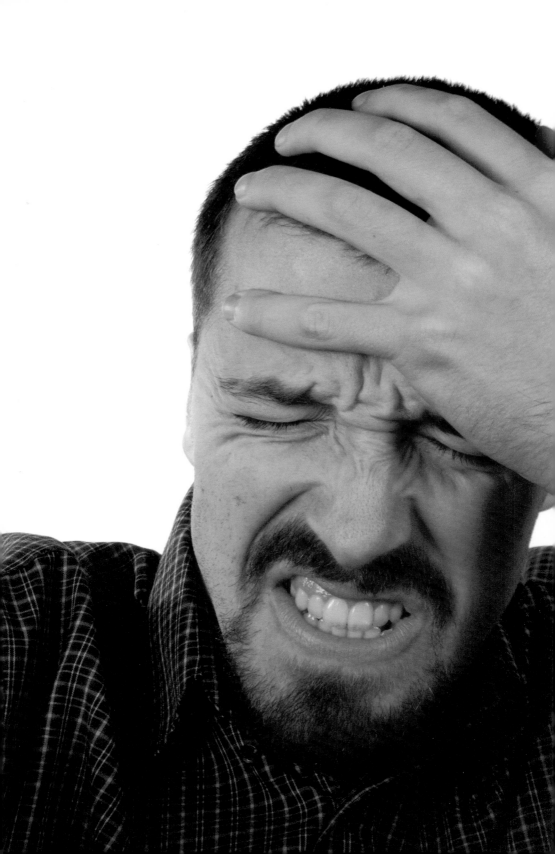

5 OxyContin

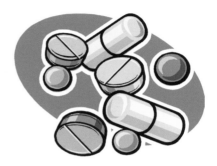

For many years, people with extreme pain could often do little more than just suffer through it—or try to at least. For them, their quality of life was severely **compromised** by an inability to manage their pain effectively. Often these were cancer patients who, besides the stress of their disease, also had to deal with debilitating pain. For others, the pain might have resulted from an injury, **bursitis**, **neuralgia**, or arthritis. In some cases, the pain was so excruciating and constant that they could only find relief when medicated so heavily they appeared "zombie-like." Though what had initially caused their pain differed, there was something these individuals shared. For many, uncontrollable pain had forced them to change their lives and in some cases, to stop doing the things they loved and enjoyed most.

In December 1995, Purdue Pharma, L.P. introduced a product to the U.S. market that promised to help thousands of people whose daily lives centered around their physical pain. (It would be introduced in Canada the following July.) OxyContin, the brand name for oxycodone hydrochloride (or oxycodone HCL), came in 10-mg, 20-mg, 40-mg, and 80-mg time-release tablets. This time-release dispersal method meant that individuals could take larger dosages. Because the medication was not released immediately, as with some opioid pain medications, the individual experienced fewer side effects when taking the larger dosages. One pill meant up to twelve hours of pain relief. It helped people escape the debilitating rollercoaster of relief and resurgence of pain accompanying shorter-acting opioids. Such benefits led to widespread use and acceptance among doctors and patients alike. Unfortunately, this meant the drug was also a relatively easy target for drug abusers and illicit drug sellers.

Oxycontin stimulates selected opioid receptors located in the CNS. Once the drug binds to these receptors, the body experiences pain relief, relaxation, slowed breathing, and a sense of euphoria. It feels better.

When taken as directed, individuals can expect to develop a dependency in a few weeks. With a physician's guidance, however, the dependency can be treated easily.

For Mary Salopek, whose story is told in the July 23, 2002, *Charlotte Observer*, the pain relief she found by using OxyContin was liberating:

Salopek, an optician, suffered persistent pain after breaking her wrist in 2000. She couldn't shower by herself. She couldn't sleep. She stopped cooking dishes she was so proud of, such as stuffed

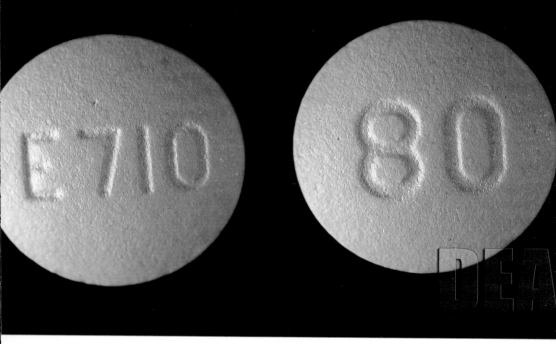

One 80-milligram tablet of OxyContin can offer hours of effective pain relief.

cabbage. She laid in bed for hours—moving even a finger induced painful spasms. A proud woman who doesn't complain, Salopek cried to her grown daughter: "It's like labor pains that never go away."

Charlotte [North Carolina] pain specialist Dr. Mark Romanoff studied her hand and wrist, so swollen he could barely make out her fingers. His diagnosis was reflex sympathetic **dystrophy**, or RSD, characterized by severe burning pain, swelling and changes in bone and skin, often occurring at an injury site. Romanoff prescribed OxyContin, as well as physical therapy and injections to block pain.

"It's like a miracle," Salopek remembered telling her daughter after taking the drug. She still takes OxyContin as prescribed. "I can't believe I suffered for so long."

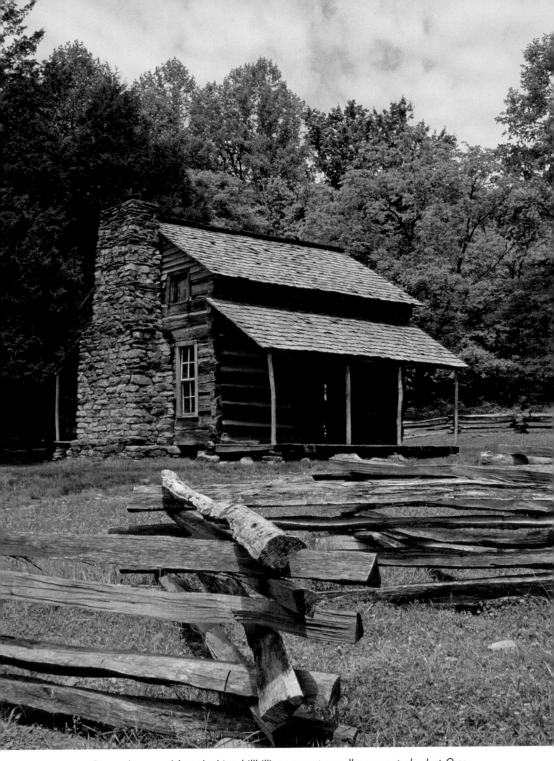

Drug abuse and Appalachian hillbillies are not usually connected—but Oxy-Contin earned itself the name "Hillbilly Heroin."

Salopek wasn't the only person who found OxyContin to be a salvation from a lifetime of pain. In just four years after it became available on the market, the sales of OxyContin in the United States reached $1 billion. Almost six million prescriptions were written for the drug in 2000. For those individuals who found relief, often for the first time in many years, OxyContin was a miracle drug. Word spread that a wonder-working pain reliever had been discovered, and its success was touted in the media. It wouldn't take long, however, before it got attention for another reason.

Hillbilly Heroin

In Lenoir, N.C., a 25-year-old mother started spending hours hunting for the drug.

Lisa, not her real name, had abused cocaine months before, but by 1999, she was trying to stay clean. Recently separated from her husband, she had a 5-year-old daughter to raise, and she wanted to remember their outings at the park or their giggles over games like Chutes and Ladders. Cocaine blurred her memory.

Then Lisa's sister started using OxyContin.

"They make you feel so good," her sister had said.

Lisa crushed and snorted a 20 milligram tablet she got from a friend. She was quickly hooked. She started spending $200 week on OxyContin, eventually pawning her wedding ring, television, CDs, even her daughter's Disney movies.

Most days, Lisa would wake up sick, and wander the streets looking for a dealer.

"It was like 10 hours of searching for four hours of a high, and then starting all over," she says.

She stopped going to church. She stopped spending time with her daughter. When she became pregnant last year, Lisa still abused the drug, even when she feared she could no longer feel the baby kick.

"I had gotten to the point where in my mind I was thinking if I lose this baby, at least I'll have something to keep me numb," she says.

The baby was born, premature but healthy. Weeks later, Lisa enrolled in a drug rehab center near Asheville, N.C.
(*Source: The Charlotte Observer*, July 23, 2002.)

Almost as quickly as individuals found relief from pain, others found alternative ways to use OxyContin, ways not intended by the manufacturer. The Charlotte Observer reported in 2002 that drug informants near Myrtle Beach, South Carolina, were telling authorities as early as 1999 about the " 'next good thing,' a tiny white pill with the marking OC." Also in 1999, law enforcement officers in York County, South Carolina, had to use the **Physicians' Desk Reference** to identify a pill they had confiscated from a teenager selling drugs out of his parents' home.

The initial reports of the nonmedical use of Oxy-Contin began coming to the attention of authorities in **Appalachia**, an area not usually thought of as being a hotbed of drug activity. In a 2003 article in the *Washington Times*, law enforcement officials were asked why they thought these rural communities were so conducive to this type of drug abuse. Many officials told reporters that

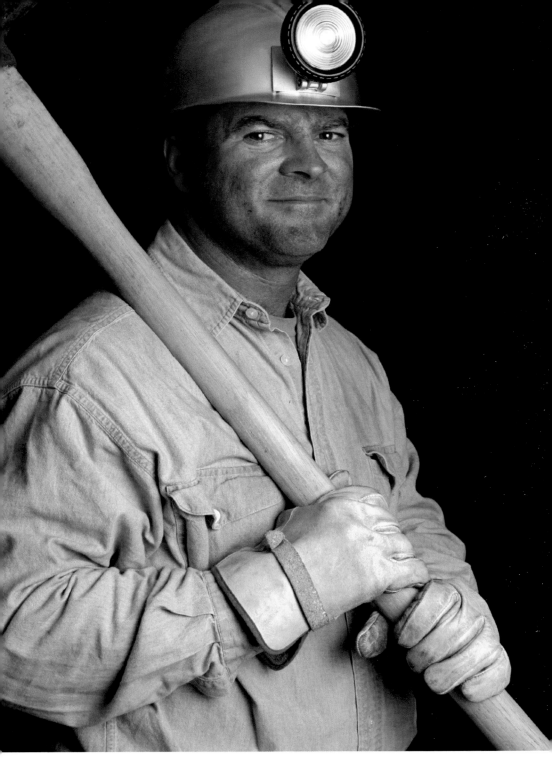

Coal miners face a variety of health risks; OxyContin offers relief for many of
their symptoms.

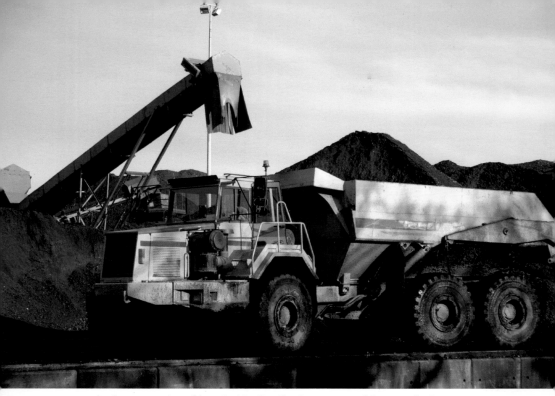

In the mountains of Appalachia, OxyContin use spread from coal mines to teenagers.

they believed the misuse of OxyContin could be traced to the coal mines in Appalachia, in particular those in Kentucky, Virginia, and West Virginia. Coal mining is dangerous, hard work and taxing on the body. For some miners, self-medicating with drugs such as OxyContin became routine just to be able to deal with the pain caused by spending long hours hunched over, sometimes almost bent in half—and in order to go back to the mine the following day to do it all over again. In the past, before certain protections were put into place, mining companies and the company doctors did whatever they believed was necessary to keep the miners working. In some cases, that included the liberal prescribing of painkillers. Just because a miner retired didn't mean the end to his pain. A lifetime of working in the mines left many retirees with injured backs, bad knees, and **black lung disease**, conditions for which OxyContin might be prescribed.

OxyContin abuse in Appalachia wasn't restricted to miners; it soon became popular with teenagers. The Washington Times article reports that some officials believe that OxyContin abuse spread to the teenage population when they snuck the pills out of their parents' and grandparents' medicine cabinets and used them to get high. Although how teens in Appalachia first started abusing OxyContin cannot be definitively determined, they did, and did so enthusiastically. The pills were in many of their parents' medicine cabinets, so the risk involved in getting the drugs was minimized. OxyContin had been prescribed by a doctor and many times paid for by government-sponsored disability programs. What this added up to in the minds of many teens was that Oxy-Contin was safer for them to take than street drugs (a common attitude of teens toward all prescription medications). Other factors that many researchers have cited as being reasons for the rapid growth of nonmedical use of OxyContin among teens included the remoteness of the region, which meant that drug enforcement officers didn't spend a lot of time looking for drug use there, and local law enforcement agencies had neither the money or the personnel to spend on drug problems; lack of access to other types of drugs; the inexpensiveness of the pills when compared to cocaine or heroin—if they could get those drugs; and that all-time favorite complaint of teens around the world: "there's nothing to do." And many of these teens were from poverty-stricken areas with little hope of achieving anything better.

Teens quickly learned that the time-release of the medication could be overridden by simply crushing the pills and then snorting the powder. Substance abuse counselor Ben Roberts is quoted in an article in the Charlotte Observer as saying that some individuals came to the clinic after melting the OxyContin pills and injecting the drug for a quicker high.

It didn't take long before authorities discovered they had a serious problem on their hands though. In 1999, drug treatment centers and hospital emergency rooms began seeing teens, pain management patients, and the casual drug user coming through their doors with similar symptoms: sweating, nausea, severe headaches—all symptoms of OxyContin withdrawal. Reports of these occurrences led law enforcement to increase their drug-related patrols. With increased drug surveillance, hardcore users moved to other areas of the South, spreading OxyContin abuse to other populations.

From Coal to Granite

While 17-year-old Ryan Curry slept, visions of OxyCotin danced in his head. Ryan was thrilled to see Oxy pills scattered under the bed, until unbearable cravings jarred him awake. Now, he could see that there were no pills. Drenched in cold sweat, Ryan's body convulsed and he began a frantic search for more OxyContin.

Ryan never thought he'd become addicted to OxyContin. . . .

Ryan, who lives in Newport, Maine, had smoked marijuana for four years before experimenting with prescription drugs. "Pot didn't have the same kick that it used to," he says. "I was bored, looking for a thrill, and trying to be cool."

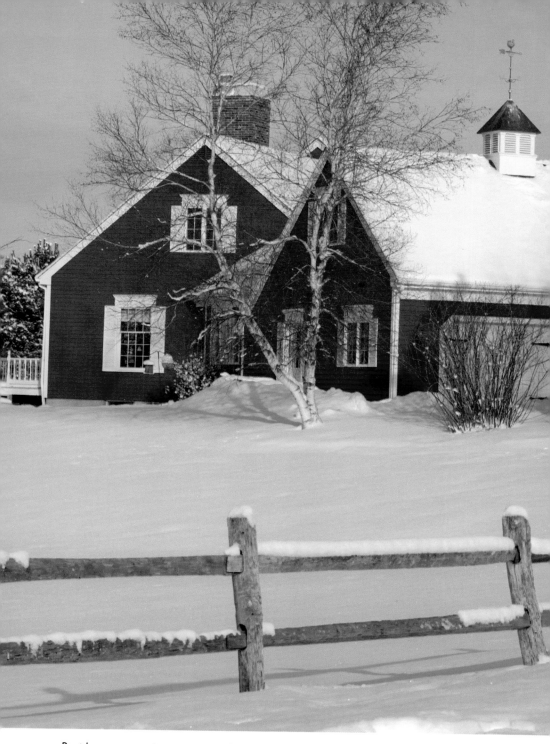

People are more apt to connect picturesque scenery than drug abuse with Maine; like the mountains of Appalachia hundreds of miles to the south, however, Maine is full of rural communities that are often poor and isolated.

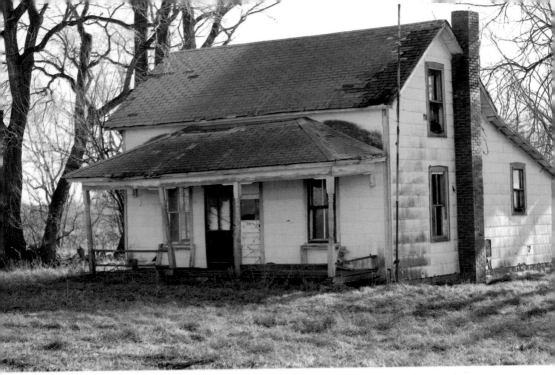

People often connect poverty and drug abuse with urban areas, but rural areas have their share of problems as well.

Ryan quickly got hooked on oxycodone. "I felt so euphoric—like I could be happy sitting in a trash can in the dark somewhere," Ryan says. . . .

Ryan quit college to work for an electrician to earn cash to buy pills. He began to use more and more OxyContin. "When I had pills, I'd feel like a king," he says. Ryan was building a physical tolerance for the drug and needed more to avoid going through withdrawal. "I'd wake up and snort 30 or 40 milligrams of Oxy—not to get high, but to feel normal, not sick." Over the next two years, Ryan went from that first 20-milligram rush to a 240-milligram-a-day habit.

(*Source:* "Crushed Dreams: Doctors Use Drugs to Heal, but in the Wrong Hands, Drugs Can Wreck Lives." *Science World,* 2004.)

They're hundreds of miles apart, but Maine and Appalachia discovered OxyContin abuse at about the same time. Maine was the first state to report a significant problem with nonmedical use of OxyContin. And, according to a 2003 article in the *Portland Press Herald*, the problem increased as the number of people described as being poor increased. Maine residents also fell victim to a false sense of security; U.S. Senator Susan Collins is quoted: "It's [prescription drug abuse] a growing crisis in most of the rural communities in our state. We've always had a sense of safety and security in Maine, and the idea that we're in the midst of an explosion of drug abuse is so contrary to our image it's hard to comprehend."

According to Maine authorities, OxyContin abuse has hit Washington County the hardest. That region is one of the poorest in the state, with industries closing and the job outlook poor. Paula Frost of Lubec Regional Medical Center tells the *Portland Press Herald*, "when you've got several industries going belly up, not even a shot at a minimum wage job, you're going to look for an escape. For generations, alcohol was an escape. Now it's OxyContin." Keya Smiley, a recovering OxyContin abuser who lives on a Native American reservation of nine hundred with a per capita income of just $14,000 a year, concurs: "Most of the people using OxyContin are like 'the hell with it. I'm going to stay high because I don't have anything.' A lot of people feel trapped."

Poverty is one thing Maine and Appalachia have in common. So are strapped law enforcement agencies. Dealers in both regions know that rural areas do not have the money to spend on drug investigations. OxyContin-related crimes other than drug dealing have increased enormously in these regions and elsewhere across the

United States. But just because they may be poor communities, doesn't mean that residents are willing to sit by and watch drugs destroy their way of life—at least not without a fight. Reverend Ronnie "Butch" Pennington, minister at the Petrey Memorial Baptist Church in Hazard, Kentucky, told the *Cincinnati Enquirer* in 2001 how his community was working to battle the OxyContin problem:

> It has been four months since 400 people attended a community meeting at his church to talk about how OxyContin has destroyed families' lives.
>
> "Kids were becoming belligerent, rebellious, stealing, lying and manipulating to support their habits," he says. "Families filed bankruptcy. Parents had their life's savings stolen by their children.
>
> "It's getting adults and children. People had a lot of hurt and pain without a lot of answers."
>
> The pages of the Hazard newspaper are filled with dozens of stories detailing the raid that locals call "Oxyfest 2001." It took nearly a full page to list the names of those indicted and the federal charges against them.
>
> So concerned was the group that it decided to create an organization called People Against Drugs. Since the October meeting at the church, the group has formed committees that will help youth and teachers recognize drug abuse. Support groups help families, and group members plan a vigil walk down the streets of Hazard.
>
> Others are monitoring drug cases in the courts.

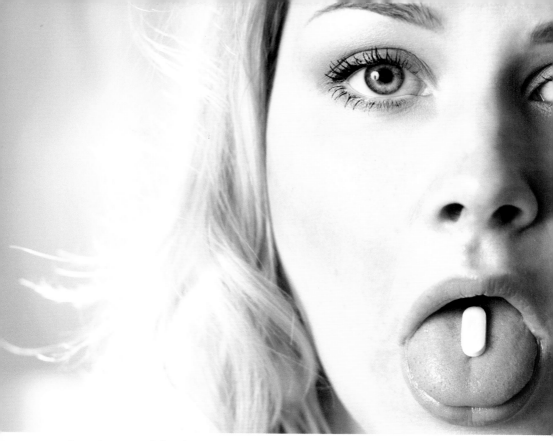

Prescription painkillers have many legitimate uses, but addiction is a real problem.

    The Rev. Mr. Pennington says the ultimate plan eventually is to provide a faith-based treatment center.

    "We are not just a watchdog group," he says. "Our attempt is to help our people."

Individuals dealing with addiction to OxyContin and other prescription painkillers can seem to get lost in the media attention on crimes related to the abuse of these drugs. But in order to reduce the related crime rates and the number of people who are losing their lives as a result of prescription painkiller addiction, effective treatment programs will have to be put in place.

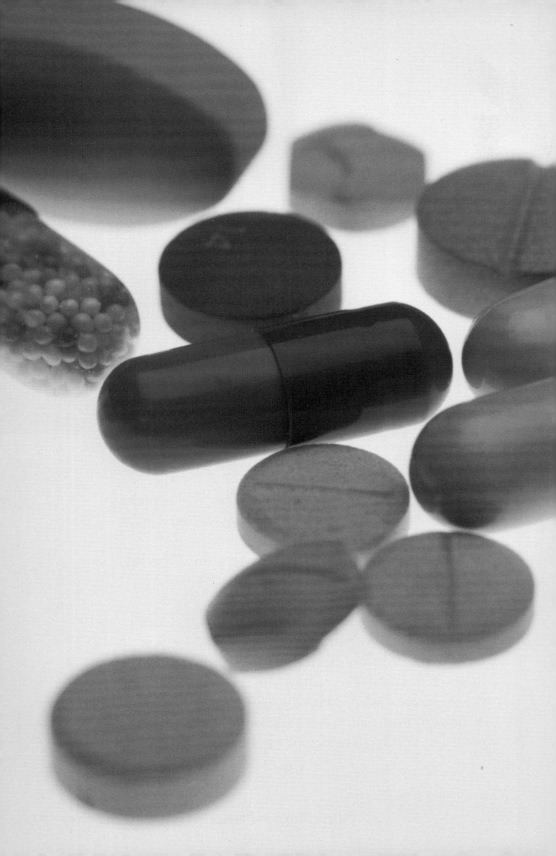

6 Treating Prescription Painkiller Addiction

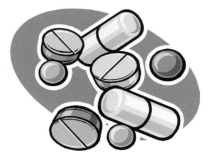

Coming off of prescription painkiller dependency or addiction is not easy and should not be done on one's own. For individuals dependent on prescription painkillers, the guidance of a health-care professional, who will generally suggest a gradual weaning from the drug through increasingly smaller dosages, can prevent or lessen withdrawal symptoms; the physical toll on the body is not as extreme as it could be. Since opioids can cause sleepiness, calmness, and constipation, those dependent or addicted to opioids may experience a "revving" up of the opposite conditions; they may experience insomnia, anxiety, and diarrhea. But the withdrawal symptoms don't stop there.

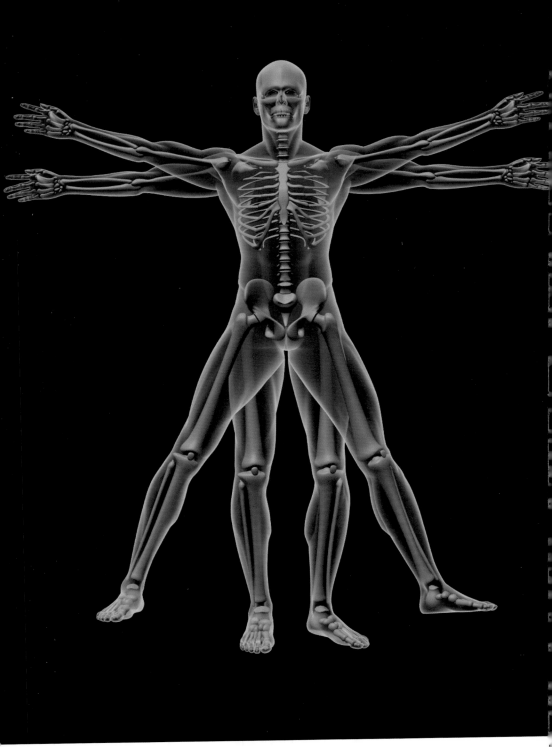

Painkiller withdrawal symptoms include muscle pain.

They can also include:

- restlessness
- sweating or chills
- muscle and joint pain
- teariness
- runny nose
- irritability
- backache
- abdominal cramps
- nausea and/or vomiting
- increased blood pressure, respiratory rate, or heart rate

In some cases, those going through withdrawal also experienced anorexia.

Breaking the bonds of prescription drug addiction can be worse than any pain someone might feel. A person addicted to OxyContin described it in an article in the *Chicago Tribune* in 2003:

> One minute I'd be freezing, the next minute I'd be hot and flailing from side to side," he said. Every minute of the day, he felt a "whole body hunger. You feel it from your little toe all the way up to your brain, like you're restless, you're closed in, you know what you need and you can't have it.
>
> You want to die—you don't know how you ended up this way. I don't know if I'm ever going to get this hunger out of my body. . . . Today, I would take any pain other than the pain of withdrawal.

The first step in overcoming addiction to prescription painkillers is the same as with every other form of addiction: admit there is a problem, that one is an addict. In some ways, this may be one of the hardest of a series of incredibly hard steps. But it is impossible to finish the journey to sobriety without taking that first step of admitting to being an addict. The person quoted above has been unable to admit to being an addict, and counselors are uncertain whether he will be successful in ending his addiction. And he's not alone. Many people with addictions complete programs without using the word "addict" to describe themselves.

The most effective method of addiction treatment involves a multidisciplinary approach—and it doesn't happen over night.

Detoxification

When one decides to break free from addiction, the body must go through a process of withdrawal to rid itself of the toxic substances of the drug. Through a medically supervised process called detoxification, the individual goes through some or all of the withdrawal symptoms listed earlier in this chapter. How long withdrawal lasts depends on how much and what type of opiate was taken. For people who are addicted to prescription painkillers, the detoxification process generally takes place in a hospital or drug treatment facility.

For someone who is dependent on prescription painkillers, this process might be enough to prevent further misuse. The person who is addicted to prescription painkillers, however, needs follow-up treatment; studies have shown that most people with addictions will return to their previous behaviors if treatment ends with detoxification. There are two primary methods of treating addiction: behavioral and *pharmacological*.

Behavioral Treatment Programs

Put simply, behavioral treatment programs teach people with addictions to change their behaviors so they are less likely to repeat those that led to addiction in the first place. Unfortunately, nothing about addiction is simple. Though behavioral treatment programs do help those with addictions find ways to avoid behaviors that can cause a relapse, they also need to help them discover what led to those behaviors initially. Cognitive-behavioral therapy helps the individuals recognize how thought patterns influence behaviors. With therapy, individuals learn how to change negative thought patterns, thereby changing behaviors. Individual and family therapy can help the person with addiction and those around her learn how to live with and as a recovering addict. Therapy can also help the addicted individual and her associates handle relapses; most people do relapse at some point during recovery.

Behavioral treatment programs also help those with addictions handle life without the prescription painkiller, including sometimes painful cravings for the drug. The individual must also learn how to deal with pain. Even if her introduction to prescription painkillers was not the result of a medical need, there may come a time when pain medications will be necessary. She needs to know how to handle that situation to lessen the possibility that she will relapse. The best treatment results are achieved when the individual practices *abstinence* from prescription painkillers.

Behavioral treatment programs often begin with a period of inpatient treatment. Depending on the length, severity, and drug of addiction, inpatient treatment can be short-term (usually a minimum of thirty days) or long-term residential. At first, some programs allow inpatients to have minimal—if any—contact with the "outside world." They concentrate on learning about themselves and their relationship with the drug. Later, family and perhaps close friends are encouraged to participate in the treatment program.

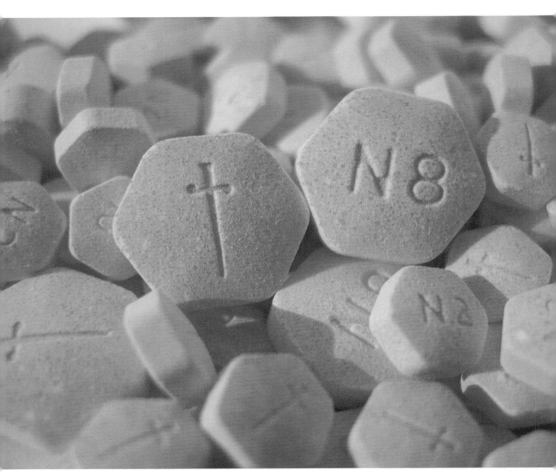

Buprenorphine is used to treat addiction to opioids. It blocks the effects of opioids on the body.

Pharmacological Treatment Programs

Medications have proven to be effective in treating addiction to opioids such as prescription pain medications. They are used in both inpatient and outpatient settings. Naltrexone, methadone, and buprenorphine are the drugs most often used in treating this addiction.

Naltrexone blocks the effects of opioids, including the sought-after highs. Methadone is a man-made drug perhaps best known as a treatment for heroin addiction. Like naltrexone, methadone blocks the effects of the opioids. It also eliminates withdrawal symptoms in those going off of the opioids, and reduces cravings for the drugs. The newest component in the pharmacological arsenal is buprenorphine, approved by the FDA in 2002. Buprenorphine can be administered by a certified doctor in an office setting, negating the need for inpatient status or trips to a drug clinic or hospital to receive ongoing treatment. Its effects are long lasting, and it is less likely to cause respiratory distress than other medications used in the treatment of prescription painkiller addiction. Although buprenorphine was tested for ten years before receiving FDA approval, its widespread use is too new to determine its long-term efficacy.

Most treatment programs use a combination of behavioral treatment and pharmacological methods. Individuals are also encouraged to supplement their programs with support groups such as Narcotics Anonymous.

Narcotics Anonymous

Based on the twelve-step program of Alcoholics Anonymous (AA), Narcotics Anonymous (NA) helps those addicted to prescription painkillers stay sober in the outside world. The first NA meetings were held in the early 1950s in Los Angeles, California. As found on its Web site (www.na.org), the organization described itself this way in its first publication:

> NA is a nonprofit fellowship or society of men and women for whom drugs had become a major problem. We . . . meet regularly to help each other stay clean. . . . We are not interested in what or how much you used . . . but only in what you want to do about your problem and how we can help.

In the more than fifty years since, NA has grown into one of the largest organizations of its kind. Today, groups are located all over the world, and its books and pamphlets are published in thirty-two languages. No matter where the group is located, each chapter is based on the twelve steps first formulated in AA:

1. We admitted we were powerless over drugs—that our lives had become unmanageable.
2. Came to believe that a Power greater than ourselves could restore us to sanity.
3. Made a decision to turn our will and our lives over to the care of God as we understand Him.
4. Made a searching and fearless moral inventory of ourselves.
5. Admitted to God, and to our selves, and to another human being the exact nature of our wrongs.
6. We're entirely ready to have God remove all these defects of character.
7. Humbly asked Him to remove our shortcomings.

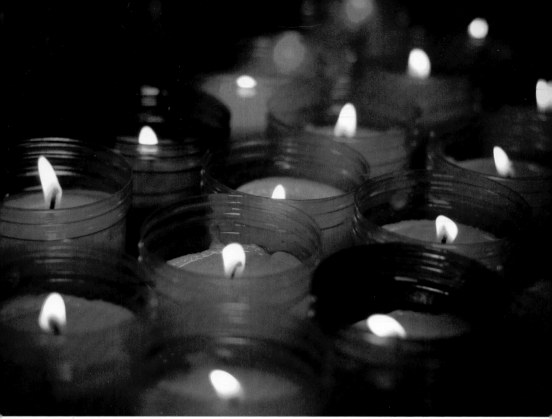

The Twelve Steps encourage those with addictions to seek strength from prayer and faith.

8. Made a list of all persons we had harmed, and became willing to make amends to them all.
9. Made direct amends to such people wherever possible, except when to do so would injure them or others.
10. Continued to take personal inventory and when we were wrong promptly admitted it.
11. Sought through prayer and meditation to improve our conscious contact with God as we understand Him, praying only for knowledge of His will for us and the power to carry that out.
12. Having had a spiritual awakening as the result of these steps, we tried to carry this message to drug addicts and to practice these principles in all our affairs.

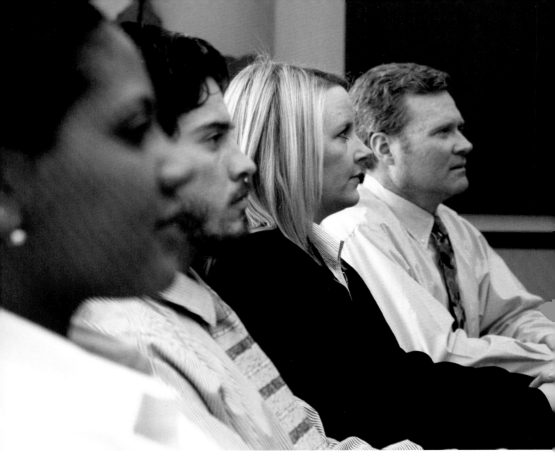

Through NA, those with addictions find help and support by meeting with others who share their problems.

Though attendance at and participation in NA meetings will not guarantee a recovery free from temptation and relapse, they can play an important role in staying sober.

Finding Help

Maine has one of the highest rates of OxyContin and other prescription painkiller addictions in the country. In the entire state, however, there are only three intensive outpatient treatment sites for children, and fewer than thirty-five residential treatment beds. Most hospitals in Maine aren't equipped for the special care that might be needed when someone is going through detoxification. In 2003, the Fordham Institute, which monitors health care, education, and income in the United States, ranked Maine thirty-sixth in the nation for treating drug- and alcohol-addicted teens.

Unfortunately, Maine isn't alone in finding it difficult to treat those with addictions who seek treatment. Other areas hit hard by prescription painkiller addiction, such as Appalachia, also have a difficult time. Limited resources and increased need have combined for what some areas is an unbeatable foe in the fight against opioid addiction. So, particularly in areas where the need is the greatest and incomes the lowest, those who are able often must travel hundreds of miles away from home to get treatment, adding additional stressors to an already trying situation.

Part of the problem lies in the fact that many North Americans don't really understand this addiction. In 2006, the U.S. National Survey of Painkiller Dependence and Treatment found that:

- 46 percent of those surveyed did not understand that painkiller abuse is as harmful as heroin abuse in terms of how it affects the body.
- 37 percent of Americans knew personally someone who abused painkillers.
- Of those surveyed who knew someone abusing painkillers, more than 20 percent reported that the abuser was a coworker.
- More than half (54 percent) of those surveyed didn't know that painkiller addiction was a medical disease.

- Survey respondents were most familiar with 12-step, abstinence, and hospital-based treatment programs; only 4 percent volunteered that medical treatment for painkiller addiction is available in doctors' offices.

The U.S. government is battling its citizens' ignorance about this growing problem with a Senate symposium on painkiller addiction treatment. Senator Orrin Hatch, one of the symposium's sponsors, stated:

Just as depression came out of the closet when it was recognized as a treatable brain disease, so should opioid dependence. The results we will present at the Senate Symposium underscore the findings of this national attitudinal survey. Clearly, education is the key to increasing awareness and opening up sufficient in-office medical treatment opportunities to help opioid-dependent people manage their disease discreetly and effectively.

New Lives

Living life without the drugs isn't always easy, but most find their new sober lives better, as noted in an interview with *Science World:*

[Dr. Jeffrey Frankenheim, a pharmacologist at the NIDA] explains, "When a person comes off the drug [OxyContin] and the brain starts coming back to normal, it can feel like a rebirth."
"True," says Ryan, who sometimes feels like a beginner in his own life. "I cry at movies I've seen before. Yesterday, I put a grape in my mouth and

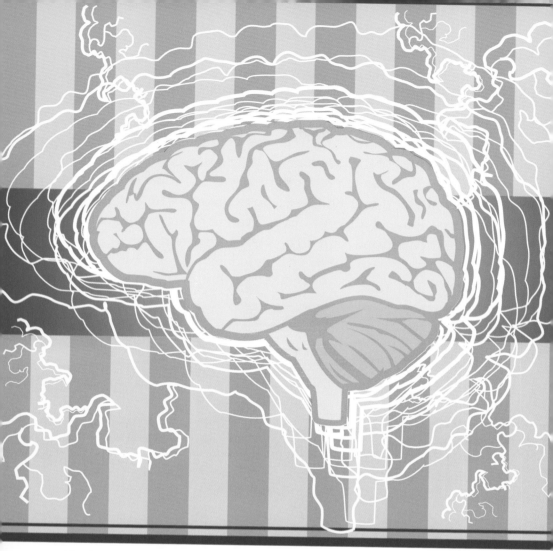

Like depression, opioid dependence is a treatable brain disease.

spit it out because it tasted more bitter than I remembered.

"I feel sad that I lost those years of my life and would give anything to get them back," Ryan says. "But now I have a life other than drugs. I'm taking college classes. I have clean friends and support. . . . I actually feel. . . . That's a big change."

Because the best "cure" is prevention, and it's better not to have to fight for those few rehabilitation resources that are available, efforts are being made to increase awareness of the problem of prescription painkiller abuse. Federal and state programs have created educational materials so young children can be taught the dangers of drug abuse of all kinds. Even Purdue Pharma, the makers of OxyContin, joined the fight to prevent abuse. They created an ad campaign, including school posters and

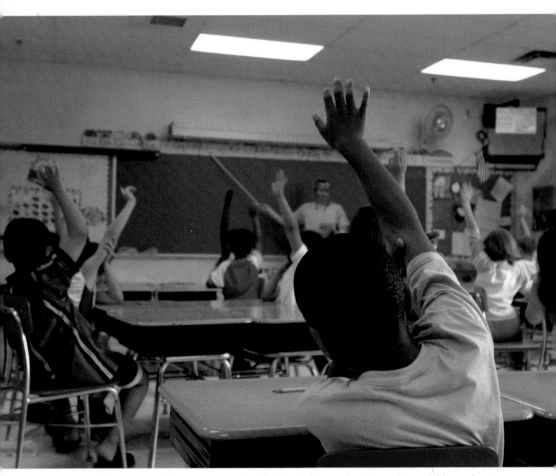

Elementary classrooms may be the best place to begin teaching children about the dangers of painkiller abuse.

classroom materials, warning about the dangers of prescription drug abuse. The posters pulled no punches, with text such as "Picking your nose at lunch does not count as dessert and *spastic* shaking caused by abusing prescription drugs is creepy," and to describe side effects of prescription drug abuse, imagery of "explosive diarrhea" and "blowing chunks."

On a grassroots level, teenagers in Whitesburg, Kentucky, weren't willing to wait for adults to do something to convince children and other teens to stay off of OxyContin. Working with Appalshop, a cultural center, they produced a documentary about the perils of OxyContin abuse. The documentary, *Because of OxyContin*, featured real-life abusers of the drug telling personal stories of how abusing the drug affected their lives. Included in the documentary was a woman from southwest Virginia who blamed the drug for her losing a child, contracting hepatitis, and possibly becoming infected with HIV.

While governments and people work to help those affected by and those who might become affected by prescription painkiller abuse, the legal community also does what it can to combat the problem.

Clifford A. Bernstein, medical director of the Waismann Method, a way of treating opiate addiction, offers parents ten suggestions on preventing prescription painkiller addiction in their children:

1. *Face the facts.* Denial can prevent you from recognizing a real problem at home. Among youths and adults, non-medical use of prescription painkillers ranked second only to marijuana in illicit drug use according to the 2002 National Survey on Drug Use and Health.

2. *Acknowledge it's all relative.* Legal or not, prescription painkillers are just as harmful as street drugs. Prescription painkillers like oxycodone are synthetic . . . opiates, the family of drugs from which heroin is derived.

3. *Keep an eye out for the graduate.* Children as young as 13–15 years old can easily graduate from abusing OxyContin (a legal opiate drug) to abusing heroin (an illegal opiate drug). The two drugs have similar effects, therefore attracting the same abuse population.

4. *Leverage what's newsworthy.* Take advantage of incidents in the news to talk to your family about painkillers. Recently, a teen in Texas was sentenced to probation for providing painkillers to a friend that died from a resulting overdose. Making an example of a story like this helps to discourage teens from trying drugs.

5. *Don't assume it can't be you.* You're not necessarily in the clear if your teen is head cheerleader or the class president. Not all kids who abuse prescription drugs are dark, depressed, and troubled. Drug use has become increasingly frequent among a variety of groups of young people.

6. *Beware of emotional rollercoasters.* Changes in a person's normal behavior can be a sign of dependency. Shifts in energy, mood, and concentration

may occur as everyday responsibilities become secondary to the need for the relief the prescription provides. Other signs to look for are social withdrawal, desensitized emotions (indifference or disinterest in things that previously brought them pleasure) and increased inactivity.

7. *Watch out for going grunge.* Personal hygiene may diminish as a result of a drug addiction. Significant weight loss may occur, and glazed eyes may indicate an underlying problem.

8. *Become a micro manager.* If your teen is prescribed a pain-relieving medication, closely monitor the dosage and frequency the drug is ingested. Also, if you or your spouse is prescribed a prescription painkiller, be sure to keep it out of your children's reach and dispose of any extras once you no longer need it.

9. *Play it smart.* Listen carefully when your doctor or pharmacist gives instructions for a drug for a family member. Provide your doctor with a complete medical history so he or she is aware of other medications being taken and can prevent a negative interaction. Finally, never increase dosage or the frequency of taking a medication without consulting your physician.

10. *Trust your instincts.* If you suspect that a family member is abusing prescription drugs, consult his or her doctor or seek professional help right away. Medical professionals can refer you to treatment programs but the most important thing is to seek help in a timely manner.

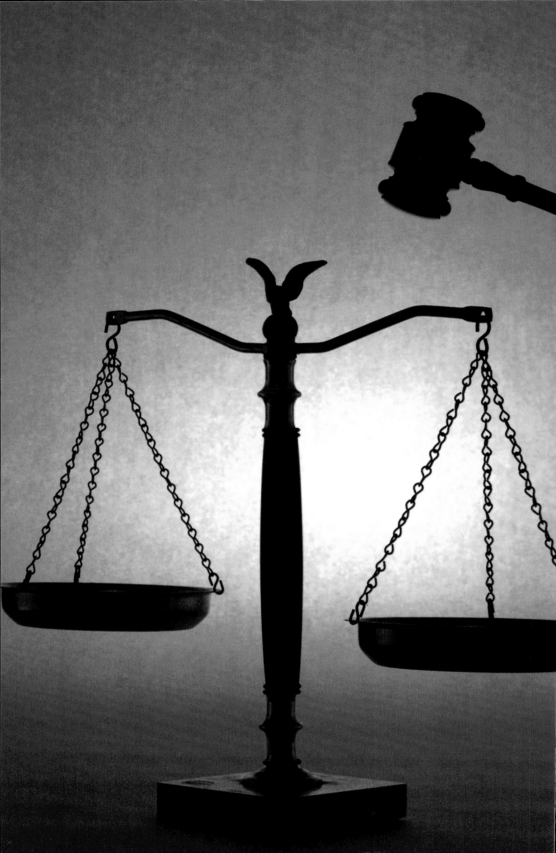

7 The Law and Prescription Painkillers

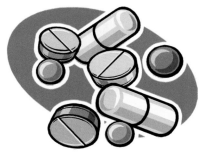

In a 2003 article in the *Portland Press Herald*, William Clark, the sheriff of Hancock County, Maine, explains his dilemma: "I only have six full-time deputies for a county of 35,000 people. I can't afford to have someone exclusively assigned to drug investigations, and the dealers out there know it."

An article in the *Washington Times* of September 2, 2003, quotes Thomas P. Lesnak, an agent with the federal Bureau of Alcohol, Tobacco, Firearms, and Explosives:

> One of the biggest problems is that when any law-enforcement officer pulls a car over and finds a prescription pill bottle in some guy's pocket, that officer ends up giving it back to the guy if it has his name on it. Maybe that officer will write the guy a speeding ticket or whatever. If it had been a gram of cocaine valued at $100 in the guy's pocket . . . he would be in jail, with felony charges.

These two officers epitomize the difficulties voiced by many in law enforcement working hard to make a dent in the problem of prescription painkiller abuse. Too few financial and personnel resources means that in some locations, dealers are fairly free to act at will. These are also the areas where abuse is most common. The ATF officer's hands are tied. As long as the prescription is in the driver's hand, as in the example quoted, there's nothing he can do. Unless the officer catches the driver in the act of illegally selling the pills, he's free to go.

Meanwhile, the number of crimes surrounding prescription painkillers such as OxyContin has increased dramatically. In 2002, the *Charlotte Observer* reported that a man in Myrtle Beach, South Carolina, robbed a pharmacy at gunpoint, but he didn't want money; he demanded OxyContin. A former high school teacher in Concord, North Carolina, was arrested and charged with attempting to hire a hit man to murder individuals who still owed him money for OxyContin. In Columbus County, North Carolina, thirty-two people were accused of selling their personal Medicaid cards to drug dealers, who then billed the state for OxyContin prescriptions. According to a 2002 report by the Office of National Drug Control Policy, most OxyContin-related crimes were robbery, burglary, larceny, and other property crimes. The DEA has reported, however, that gunrunning and the sale of stolen guns has played a role in financing drug dealing of prescription painkillers.

Law enforcement is not only targeting the street dealers. The DEA is also going after doctors who write phony prescriptions for painkillers and the unscrupulous pharmacists who fill them. In Operation Cotton Candy, which took place in 2003 in Virginia, doctors were found who signed prescriptions for large amounts of OxyContin

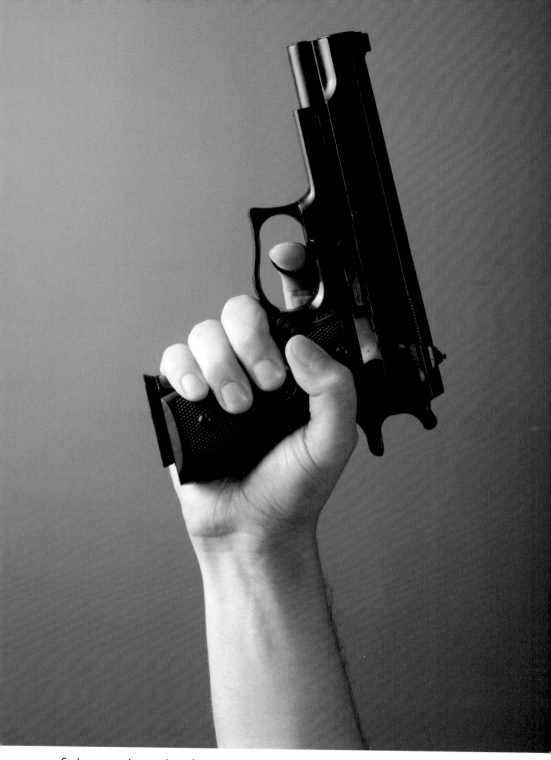

Stolen guns play a role in financing prescription painkiller sales.

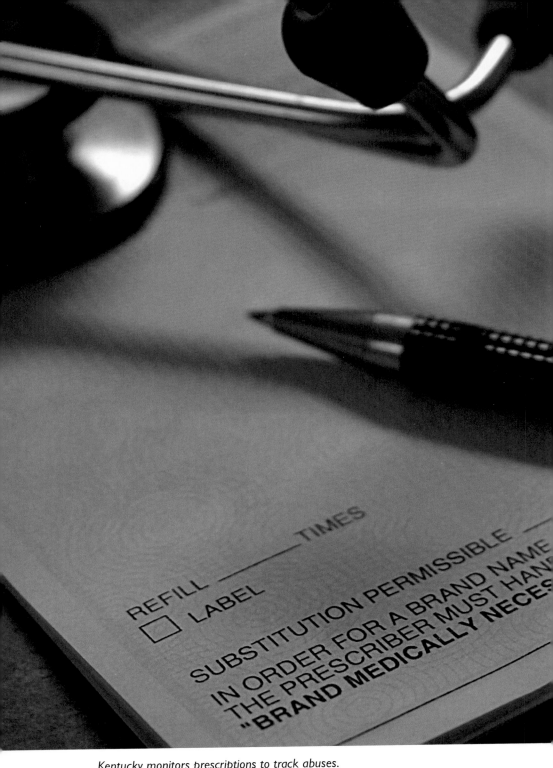

REFILL _____ TIMES

☐ LABEL

SUBSTITUTION PERMISSIBLE

IN ORDER FOR A BRAND NAME

THE PRESCRIBER MUST HAN[

"BRAND MEDICALLY NECES

Kentucky monitors prescriptions to track abuses.

to people who turned around and sold the pills on the black market. But medical professionals' involvement in the illegal distribution of prescription painkillers is not limited to Virginia. All over the country, ethical pharmacists alert law enforcement officials when customers start showing up with a large number of painkiller prescriptions from a particular doctor. In some areas, the DEA has set up telephone hotlines for patients themselves to report doctors they feel are overprescribing OxyContin.

There's only so much law enforcement can do in their campaign to get illegally obtained prescription painkillers off the street.

The Legislature

Once stories about prescription painkiller abuse became known to the media, legislatures across the country began working to create and toughen laws pertaining to illegal buying and selling of prescription medications. In 1999, Kentucky became the first state to establish a prescription-monitoring program; several states have since adopted similar programs. The Kentucky legislature has acted to make the program more efficient and searches more timely by approving police use of the Kentucky All Schedule Prescription Electronic Reporting System (KASPER) to track abuses by location rather than initiating a request based on a single incident. Police agencies working on regional investigations can share the information from KASPER, rather than each department filing a separate request to get the information. Purdue Pharma, maker of OxyContin, has contributed funding toward the creation of a prescription-tracking program available to states.

Though buying controlled substances without a prescription is a federal offense, it is a law that is difficult to enforce when it comes to Internet sales. Often it is impossible for authorities to determine where these businesses are located. Many are located in Canada, Mexico, or offshore, which makes it difficult—if not impossible—for authorities to regulate. In 2006, the House Government Reform Committee held hearings on a bill requiring such Web sites to identify their locations as well as the names of doctors and pharmacists affiliated with the sites. The bill would also ban any sales made without an in-person consultation with a doctor and a valid prescription.

The White House Office of National Drug Control Policy has ordered federal agencies with antidrug programs to develop new strategies to combat prescription drugs' abuse and illegal marketing. According to director John P. Walters, "We don't want to wait until we get what we had with the crack epidemic. Hopefully we're a little bit earlier in the process."

Under the new plan, the FDA and DEA would have primary responsibility for the focus on prescription drugs. The Office of National Drug Control Policy asked the FDA to improve labeling for the most-often abused prescription drugs. Closure of online businesses, including pharmacies, selling drugs without prescriptions would be the responsibility of the DEA.

Meanwhile, some citizen groups feel the government needs to take a still tougher stance. For instance, the Public Citizens' Health Research Group believes that the FDA should totally ban the painkiller Darvocet and its chemical cousins. The Associated Press reported on March 2, 2006, that the group contends the drug caused more than 2,100 accidental deaths between 1981 and

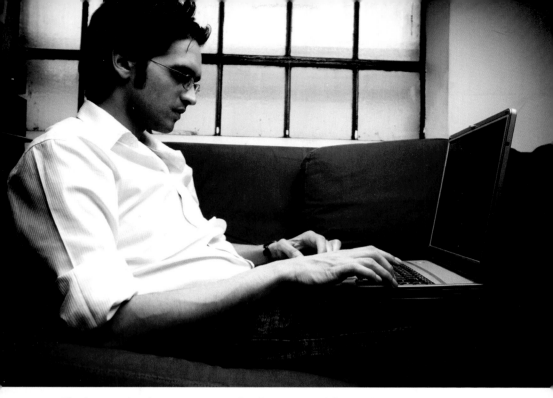

The Internet has become a source for obtaining painkillers without prescriptions. The DEA is trying to close these online pharmacies.

1999, and that it has also been used by thousands more to commit suicide. Public Citizen petitioned the FDA to ban propoxyphene, the main ingredient in Darvon and Darvocet, saying it carries unacceptable risk for a relatively weak painkiller. Although propoxyphene has been sold legally in the United States since 1957, Public Citizen has been trying to get it banned ever since 1978. "This a black-and-white example of a drug where its risks far outweigh its benefits," said Public Citizen's Sidney Wolfe. "There's no excuse for this drug to be around." In 2005, regulators in the United Kingdom decided on a phased ban on the drug, but in the United States, 23 million prescriptions for propoxyphene-based drugs continue to be written each year.

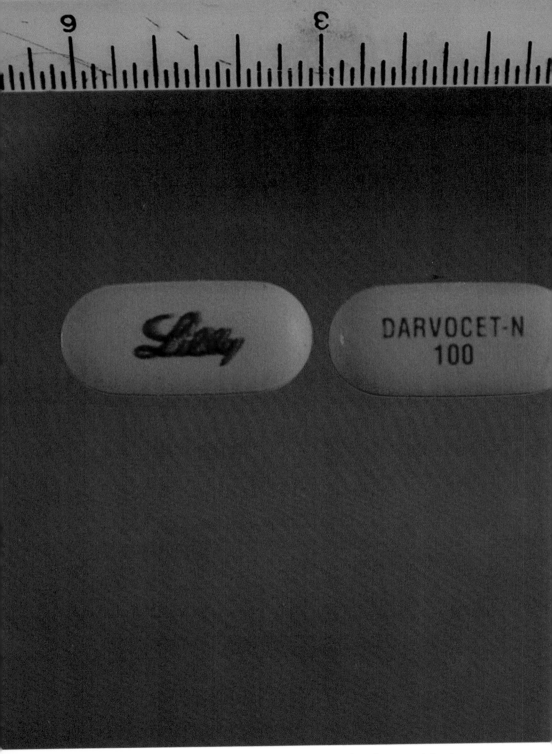

Darvocet contains propoxyphene, a painkiller that has the potential to be abused.

As the government, law enforcement, and honest doctors and pharmacists work together, they hope they will be able to stem the tide of prescription painkiller abuse. Though some people have called for the pulling from the marketplace drugs such as OxyContin, the answer may not be that simple.

Ultimately, some say, the argument goes back to Western culture's perception of pain: Is it a meaningless and unpleasant experience that must be medically relieved at all costs? Or do human beings have spiritual and mental abilities that might allow them to manage their pain in other ways?

There are many possible answers to these questions. After all, these medications have an important role to play in pain management and in improving the quality of life for millions of individuals. Many people insist that painkillers can be used responsibly to help rather than harm.

What do you think?

Rod Colvon, author of *Prescription Drug Addiction: The Hidden Epidemic*, recommends that patients take a more active role in their health care by following these steps:

- When prescribed any drug, ask your doctor if it's addictive. "Many people get hooked on prescription drugs merely because the don't realize the drug they're on is habit-forming," explains Colvin. "By knowing this from the outset, patients can avoid becoming addicts through sheer ignorance."
- If your family has a history of drug addiction or alcoholism, tell your doctor; it may mean that you're not a good candidate for the more addictive drugs or that you should be monitored more closely.
- If at any point you feel your doctor is not taking the time to fully understand your problems or explain your treatment and its side effects, insist on seeing a physician who will—if possible, someone who specializes in pain management, anxiety disorders, or addiction.
- If the drug you're being prescribed is habit forming, ask your doctor, "How quickly could I develop a dependence?" If you're on these drugs for this amount of time or longer, discuss with your doctor how you should taper off the drug to prevent withdrawal symptoms.
- While you're taking these drugs, monitor yourself for signs of addiction. Colvin suggests keeping these questions in mind: Have you ever felt that the amount of the drug you're prescribed isn't working as well as it used to? Do you experience more than just symptom relief on the drug, such as a feeling of excitement, or a "high"? Do you feel that you can perform certain tasks or activities (like driving in traffic or socializing at parties) only with the medication? If you answer yes to any of these questions, this may be a sign that you should broach the subject of addiction with your doctor.
- While on these drugs, ask three friends or family members to keep an eye on you as well. Say to them, "I'm on a medication that's potentially addictive. Can you tell me if you notice my personality changing over time—say, if I'm acting too happy, or more remote or irritable than usual?" The less secrecy and shame you have about using these drugs, the more likely you are to get help if you need it, says Colvin. "Most people understand alcoholism," he says. "But when an addict's drug of choice comes from a doctor, there's a lot more confusion. People think, Maybe she's supposed to be taking these. The more people who know that prescription drugs can be a problem, the faster we can stop this epidemic of addiction.

Glossary

abstinence: Restraint from indulging in a desire for something.

advocacy: Active verbal support for a cause or position.

alchemist: Someone who practices an early, unscientific form of chemistry, seeking to turn base metals into gold and to discover a life-prolonging medicine.

alkaloid: A nitrogen-containing alkaline compound found in plants and used in medicines, drugs, or as a poison.

Appalachia: The U.S. region that includes the southern Appalachian Mountains, extending from southwestern Pennsylvania through West Virginia and parts of Kentucky and Tennessee to northwestern Georgia.

black lung disease: A lung disease caused by the long-term inhalation of coal dust; anthracosis.

bursitis: An inflammation of a fluid-filled sac of the body, especially at the elbow, knee, or shoulder joint.

compromised: Impaired the functioning of something or someone.

compulsive: Driven by an irresistible inner force to do something.

consensus: General or widespread agreement among all members of a group.

contraindications: Reasons for not taking a medication due to possible adverse reactions.

controlled substances: Drugs subject to legal controls.

cytoplasm: The chemical compounds and structures within a plant or animal cell excluding the nucleus.

dispersed: Scattered in different directions.

doctor shop: To go from doctor to doctor getting prescriptions.

dystrophy: Progressive degeneration of a body tissue.

efficacy: Ability to produce the necessary or desired results.

enigma: Something not easily explained or understood.

euphoria: Extreme joy or sense of well-being.

gastrointestinal: Relating to the stomach and intestines.

neuralgia: Intermittent and often severe pain in a part of the body that a particular nerve runs through.

neuropsychological: Relating to the influence of the nervous system on psychology.

neurotransmitters: Chemicals that carry messages between different nerve cells.

pharmacological: Relating to the science or study of drugs.

Physicians' Desk Reference: A book that contains the information provided in the package inserts with prescription drugs.

potent: Powerful.

probation: The action of suspending the sentence of a convicted offender and giving the offender freedom during good behavior while being supervised by a probation officer.

purgatives: Drugs or other substances that cause evacuation of the bowels.

quadriplegics: People who cannot move all four limbs or the body below the neck.

quantified: Expressed by number.

radiate: To spread out from a central point.

scirrhus: A cancerous tumor that is hard and fibrous.

spastic: Used to describe a condition characterized by a sudden muscle contraction.

strychnine: A bitter, white, poisonous alkaloid.

synthesized: Combined separate things into a new whole.

Western: Typical of countries whose cultures and societies are greatly influenced by traditions rooted in Greek and Roman culture and Christianity.

Further Reading

Durham, Michael. *Painkillers and Tranquilizers*. Portsmouth, N.H.: Heinemann, 2003.

Glass, George. *Narcotics: Dangerous Painkiller*. New York: Rosen, 2001.

Harris, Nancy (ed.). *Opiates*. Farmington Hills, Mich.: Thomson Gale, 2005.

Lawton, Sandra Augustyn (ed.). *Drug Information for Teens: Health Tips About the Physical and Mental Effects of Substance Abuse: Including Information About Marijuana, Inhalants, Club Drugs, Stimulants, Hallucinogens, Opiates, Prescription and Over-the-Counter Drugs*. Detroit, Mich.: Omnigraphics, 2006.

Pinsky, Drew, Stephanie Brown, Robert J. Meyers, and William White. *When Painkillers Become Dangerous: What Everyone Needs to Know About OxyContin and Other Prescription Drugs*. Center City, Minn.: Hazelden Publishing, 2004.

For More Information

Center for Drug Evaluation and Research (information about Oxy-Contin Tablets)
www.fda.gov/cder/drug/infopage/oxycontin

Family Guide
family.samhsa.gov/talk/painkillers.aspx

Parenting Teens
www.parentingteens.com/prescription_drug_abuse.html

Teens Health
kidshealth.org/teen/drug_alcohol/drugs/prescription_drug_abuse.html

Waismann Method Advanced Treatment of Opiate Dependency
www.opiates.com

The Web sites listed on this page were active at the time of publication. The publisher is not responsible for Web sites that have changed their addresses or discontinued operation since the date of publication. The publisher will review and update the Web-site list upon each reprint.

Bibliography

Bhatt, Sanjay. "OxyContin Maker's Gross Ads Seek to Steer Teens from Pill Abuse." *Palm Beach Post*, November 8, 2001.

Cenziper, Debbie. "OxyContin: Misuse, Overuse of Drug Blamed for Crime, Shattered Lives and Deaths." *Charlotte Observer*, July 23, 2002.

Colvin, Rod. *Prescription Drug Addiction: The Hidden Epidemic*. New York: Addicus, 2001.

Cousins, Norman. *Anatomy of an Illness*. New York: W. W. Norton, 2005.

D'Angelo, Laura. "Crushed Dreams: Doctors Use Drugs to Heal, but in the Wrong Hands, Drugs Can Wreck Lives." *Science World*, March 8, 2004.

Goetz, Kristina. "The Faces of OxyContin." *Cincinnati Enquirer*, February 25, 2001.

Graham, Judith. "Painful Rehab Follows Addiction to Painkillers." *Chicago Tribune*, October 19, 2003.

Morris, David B. *The Culture of Pain*. Berkeley: University of California, 1993.

National Institute on Drug Abuse. Research Report: Prescription Drugs Abuse and Addiction. Washington, D.C.: U.S. Department of Health and Human Services, National Institutes of Health, 2005.

Taylor, Guy. "OxyContin Abuse Becomes Scourge for Teens in Rural Areas." *Washington Times*, September 2, 2003.

"Teens' Video Focuses on OxyContin's Horrors." *Cincinnati Post*, September 7, 2001.

"Treating Opiate Addiction, Part I: Detoxification and Maintenance." http://www.health.harvard.edu/newsweek/Treating_opiate_addiction.

Walsh, Barbara. "New Rite of Rural Poverty: Prescription Drug Addiction Has Reached Rates One Would Never Expect in Maine, with the Poorest Seeing the Worst of It." *Portland Press Herald*, December 17, 2003.

Index

Picture Credits

Forca–Fotolia: p. 66
Harvey, Chris–Fotolia: p. 30
Hasegawa, Naomi–Fotolia: p. 13
iStockphotos: pp. 10, 90, 98
    Cornell, Cyrus: p. 110
    Harvey, Chris: p. 18
    Jones, Sandy: p. 34
    Kaulitzki, Sebastian: p. 39
    Knape, Satu: p. 86
    Lewis, David H.: p. 15
    Louie, Nancy: p. 102
    Nichols, Greg: p. 82
    Panosian, S. Greg: p. 77
    Romain, Malcolm: p. 81
    Scivally, Shawn: p. 50
    Simon, Robert: p. 85
    Soler, Ferran Traite: p. 97
    Tanir, Kutay: p. 109
    Torquato, Vincent: p. 101
    Trojanowksa, Gabriela: p. 16
    Wilton, Dan: p. 113
    Young, Lisa F.: p. 78
Jupiter Images: p. 88
Koval, Vasiliy–Fotolia: p. 8
Motrenko, Alexander–Fotolia: p. 25
Slusarczyk, Marek–Fotolia: p. 70
Snover, JoAnn–Fotolia: p. 26
U.S. Drug Enforcement Agency: pp. 68, 74, 94, 114
U.S. National Library of Medicine: p. 28
Van Den Berg, Simone–Fotolia: pp. 57, 64
Vanovitch, Lisa–Fotolia: p. 60
Webdata: p. 106
Zidar, Dusan–Fotolia: p. 48

To the best knowledge of the publisher, all other images are in the public domain. If any image has been inadvertently uncredited, please notify Harding House Publishing Service, Vestal, New York 13850, so that rectification can be made for future printings.

Author and Consultant Biographies

Author

Ida Walker is a graduate of the University of North Iowa in Cedar Falls, and has done graduate work at Syracuse University. The author of several nonfiction books, she currently lives in Upstate New York.

Series Consultant

Jack E. Henningfield, Ph.D., is a professor at the Johns Hopkins University School of Medicine, and he is also Vice President for Research and Health Policy at Pinney Associates, a consulting firm in Bethesda, Maryland, that specializes in science policy and regulatory issues concerning public health, medications development, and behavior-focused disease management. Dr. Henningfield has contributed information relating to addiction to numerous reports of the U.S. Surgeon General, the National Academy of Sciences, and the World Health Organization.